Springer

Tokyo
Berlin
Heidelberg
New York
Barcelona
Budapest
Hong Kong
London
Milan
Paris
Santa Clara
Singapore

M. Shimizu (Ed.)

Recent Progress in
Child and Adolescent Psychiatry

With 17 Figures

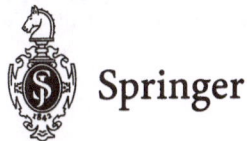 Springer

Masayuki Shimizu, M.D., Ph.D.
Director in Chief
Mie Prefectural Asunaro Hospital
   for Child and Adolescent Psychiatry
1-12-3 Shiroyama, Tsu-si, Mie 514, Japan

ISBN-13: 978-4-431-70172-9   e-ISBN-13: 978-4-431-68525-8
DOI: 10.1007/978-4-431-68525-8

Printed on acid-free paper

Typesetting: Best-set Typesetter Ltd., Hong Kong

Preface

We are nearing the end of the twentieth century, a period that Ellen Key had earnestly hoped would be a century for children. Key was a philosopher who took a hard look at the future of Sweden around the beginning of this century when it was a developing nation rapidly becoming industrialized. Many countries, including Japan, have shared Key's hopes that children would become the leaders in a century filled with possibilities. In sharp contrast to those bright expectations, however, the century has often brought very hard times for children and adolescents. The world never has seemed to focus on its children, nor has it inspired them with great hope. To the contrary, it has driven them again and again into such dangers and destruction as those incurred by merciless wars.

The professional discipline of child and adolescent psychiatry has developed in this century, especially in its latter half. As a medical field, it has made significant advances, but child and adolescent psychiatry cannot be satisfied to remain so narrowly defined. The last two letters of IACAPAP, an international academic society for child and adolescent psychiatry, stand for "Allied Professions," which means that we work in cooperation with those in other professions. What we are expected to do as professions, then, goes beyond simply treating or caring for children's disabilities or diseases. We must also be aware of our responsibilities for the healthy development of every generation in every community.

With this outlook, we decided to publish the current collection of papers on child and adolescent psychiatry and related studies. We present here what we hope will be the first in a series of forthcoming volumes. We welcome contributions as well as critical comment from our readers and professional colleagues in all parts of the world.

Masayuki Shimizu

Contents

Part 1. Developmental Disorders

Part 2. Infant Psychiatry

Part 3. School Refusals

Part 4. Neurotic Disorders

Part 5. Psychotic Disorders

Part 6. Other Fundamental Problems

Part 1

Developmental Disorders

Present Conditions and Problems at Facilities for Autistic Adults

Koji Okuno, Yasuhiko Kondo, and Nishiki Chikusa

Summary. Services for autistic adults are still not institutionally organized in Japan. Because of the urgent problems of these adults, they are now receiving training under the category of services for the mentally retarded, and there are more than 10 facilities of this type around the country. These facilities can be divided into three types according to the process of their establishment: (1) facilities promoted and organized by a group of parents; (2) facilities operated by an existing social welfare organization for the benefit of community residents; and (3) facilities established by administrative agencies or an existing social welfare organization in response to lobbying by parents and volunteers. Each facilities has its own character and its own problems according to the process of its establishment and the nature of the surrounding community. Asake Gakuen is the first specialized home for autistic adults in Japan. It was designed to be a model for facilities for the developmentally disabled that focus on autistic adults. It facilitates social independence through on-site work experience and ties with the local community. The details of the establishment of Asake Gakuen and its present condition are introduced, and its present conditions, policies and problems concerning the role of facilities for autistic adults in Japan are discussed.

Key words. Facility for autistic adults—On-site work—Association with the community—Social independence

Autistic children in Japan are still said to have "handicaps" and are excluded from the existing system because of their specific syndrome and the existence of no institutional place in the medical, educational, or social welfare system. At present, the facilities available to autistic adolescents and adults were founded in all cases by their parents. The number of these facilities has increased rapidly, so there were at least 10 institutions of this type in Japan in 1988. Because of the urgent problems of autistic adults, they receive training under the category "services for the mentally retarded." These facilities can be divided into three types according to the process of their establishment. It may be said that Asake Gakuen is included in the first type.

1. Facilities promoted and organized by a group of parents
2. Facilities operated by an existing social welfare organization for the benefit of community residents

Asake Gakuen, 1573 Komono-cho, Mie-gun, Mie 510, Japan

3. Facilities established by administrative agencies or an existing social welfare organization in response to lobbying by parents and volunteers

Each facility has its own character and its own problems according to the process of its establishment and the nature of the surrounding community. The details of the establishment of Asake Gakuen and its present condition are introduced herein, and its present conditions, policies, and problems concerning the role of facilities for autistic adults in Japan are discussed.

Establishment of Asake Gakuen

Asake Gakuen is the first specialized home for autistic adults in Japan. It was designed in 1981 to be a model for residential facilities for the developmentally disabled, focusing on autistic adults. Many residents were trained at the Mie Prefectural Child Medicine Center (Asunaro Gakuen), but there was some anxiety about their future because they must graduate at age 18. Because of this rule the parents of these adolescents have provided a residential facility.

The parents' anxieties were that (1) their children were not provided with adult-adequate residential care; (2) services for autistic adults were not supported by institutional care; and (3) the conditions at the time excluded them from any of the conventional facilities.

The preparatory committee for Asake Gakuen was formally established in 1973. The family-based group began a fund-raising campaign, and it was eventually given some private grant. Throughout their campaign the group recognized the following policies about facility management.

1. *Association with the community*: It was designed with the fundamental view that the individual could maintain a productive and useful life in the community.
2. *Voluntary life*: A situation was created that not only protected but also facilitated adult life for the individual.
3. *Work as a medium for social training*: The individual could relate to community people through a job and so could acquire realistic skills and behaviors.
4. *Consideration for individual handicaps*: The training program, techniques, and psychiatric approach were devised to accommodate special impairments.
5. *Educational movement to the community*: The program was based on the concept that the existence of handicapped people can raise a question about feelings and togetherness among all people. The establishment of our facilities provides one answer to this question.

The thoughts described here were influenced by the policy on which the therapeutic and systematic programs for autistic children and adolescents were based in Asunaro Gakuen. The family's enthusiasm has focused on social togetherness, which respects handicapped persons for their individuality and their role of society.

Present Conditions in Asake Gakuen

Population

Table 1 shows the sex and ages of our residents. The population consists of 40 individuals (male 30, female 10). The age distribution is 15 to 37 years old. In terms of

Table 1. Sex and age of 40 autistic adults.

Sex	Age (years)					Total
	15–19	20–24	25–29	30–35	35–40	
Male	6	14	5	5	0	30
Female	1	6	1	1	1	10
Total	7	20	6	6	1	40

Table 2. IQ and diagnosis of 40 autistic adults.

IQ	Autistic	Nonautistic		Total
		Psychosis	Mentally retarded	
Severely retarded	25	0	4	29
Moderately to mildly retarded	5	1	5	11
Total	30	1	9	40

the diagnosis, there were 30 autistic adolescents and adults and 10 nonautistic, developmentally disabled persons (Table 2). Their IQs range from untestable to mildly mentally retarded. Several of the moderately retarded persons also have emotional disturbances, such as thievish habits, violence, and wandering.

Eighty percent of the residents had utilized Asunaro Gakuen before becoming resident in Asake Gakuen. The remaining residents were admitted directly from their home or a special school, but most had not been provided with appropriate educational programs. The disabilities of those from special schools are milder than the problems of the persons who had attended Asunaro Gakuen. The remainder of the residents' self-help and social skills have been judged severely handicapped.

Placement of the Staff

The institution comprises two residential units with 20 residents each: Unit A and Unit B. Two staff persons in each residential unit offer night care. Placement of the staff is shown in Table 3. We have almost twice the direct-care staff members as are called for by statutory provision, but they have night duty several times during a month as well. Morever, they must hold an office in addition to providing occupational training and guidance; and they must participate in instruction about sports,

Table 3. Placement of staff.

Occupation	Statutory provision	Asake-Gakuen
Chief officer	1	1
Doctor	1	1
Nurse		2
Care staff	10	18
Facilitator		1
Dietitian		1
Office worker	1	1
Kitchen staff	4	4
Cleaner		1
Total	17	30

Table 4. Visits to neighboring hospitals, by specialty.

Specialty	1984	1985	1986
Internal medicine	117	53	57
Surgery	143	140	39
Dentistry	126	130	90
Ear, nose, throat	48	19	35
Ophthalmology	10	4	3
Dermatology	46	32	53
Gynecology	69	5	2
Psychiatry	179	233	179
Others	6	0	7
Total	744	616	465

leisure activities, learning cognitive skills, psychological assessment, and family counseling.

In the near future we hope to separate the therapeutic section from the residential one. We would rather have some professional staff and use our social resources staff for sports, leisure, and cultural activities.

Medical Care

Autistic adolescents and adults frequently experience an uncontrolled panicky response, self-injury, persistence epileptic seizures, and a lack of activity exceeding that of infants. Detailed behavioral observation and medical attention are required to alleviate these problems. Our purpose, in association with providing medical care, is to enable the individual to self-control these behavioral disorders, which interfere with daily living, working, and social activities. The medical treatment is given careful attention, with a psychiatric consultation and case conference twice in a month.

We utilize hospitals near our facility for consultations in internal medicine, surgery, and the other specialties. The numbers of such visits to these hospitals annually are shown in Table 4.

Association with the Community

Our idea for establishing the facility was not to provide a sheltered life but to promote social participation of autistic people in the community. Therefore we must provide them with various social activities (e.g., work and leisure) within the community. The placement of our facilities were determined with this thought in mind, and the site was chosen from nearly 20 proposed sites. The standards by which we selected the site included the fact that it was in a residential section and that it had favorable areas for shopping, hair-cuts, transport, and job opportunities, among others.

Initially there were many complaints from the neighborhood. However, as our residents' daily living habits have calmed down and become quiet and participation in some town events has become more frequent, others in the neighborhood have changed their opinions, and they now give a positive report of our residents. For instance, whenever they see autistic adults working, shopping, and jogging, they

Table 5. Club activities.

Club	No.	Activities
Music	10	Instrumental music, appreciation of music
Sports	9	Softball, marathon, watching baseball games
Ceramic art	8	Displays in exhibitions

express praise for the growth of the residents. With this background, it is natural that many behavioral disorders can be improved in relation to the individuals' surroundings. Concerns exist and are best dealt with keeping in mind certain principles.

1. Allow residents to join in events only after rehearsal of the activity.
2. Make contact with regional organizations and voluntary groups.
3. If there is a complaint, the staff copes with it as soon as possible.
4. Whatever the question, maintain the attitude that the residents are "handicapped individuals".

Our residents may go shopping daily, get a haircut, go to a movie theater, or visit a coffee shop—and have for some time. There are ongoing programs to facilitate going out oneself or in a small group. In a gradually stepped-up program, shop workers in the town have become willing to accept the disabilities of our residents. Therefore several persons take lessons on the piano or drum, swimming lessons, and are learning the art of flower arranging. Their leisure time is usually spent at three club activities (Table 5) and at annual events, such as travel, skiing, a summer festival, and a year-end party. Whenever these events are held, neighbors and volunteers join in and visit our facilities.

Everyday Life Program in Residential Units

Autism is primarily a combination of impaired cognitive skills and behavioral disorders. Those who are disabled have difficulty with their self-help functions in the activities of daily living (ADL). Our facilities have established the ADL programs shown in Table 6, which are aimed at individual self-actualization in the residential unit.

Autistic disorders often manifest a tendency toward patterned behaviors and have extreme dislike against change. The intent of the ADL programs is to acquire survival

Table 6. Daily programs in Asake Gakuen.

Time	Daily programs
6:30	Rise; make bed; get dressed; wash face; shave; clean room
7:00	Eat breakfast; brush teeth
8:30	Morning conference with staff
9:30	Start work[a]
12:00	Eat lunch
15:30	End work; go home (to each living unit)[a]; arrange clothes
16:00	Perform physical exercise (e.g., jog); enjoy free time
18:30	Eat evening meal; bathe; enjoy free time: watch television, read, write in diary, wash clothes, other activities
22:00	Go to bed

[a] Except on holidays.

skills. We are convinced that one of the most important points is not only the sequential aspect but the individual's situation in life. For example, the residents acquire skills for making use of the bathroom, kitchen, and other life environments. Thus we must take into account their degree of competence. It is important to use different instruction modes (e.g., oral speech, demonstration, gestures, pictures, letter cards), according to the need of the individual.

During the passage of daily living several modifications in the ADL take place if an unexpected visitor arrives or unexpected business takes place. As soon as an autistic person moves into our facility, he or she frequently has a panicky response. To put him or her at ease we describe the daily programs (eating and bathing) or the television channels as frequently as is needed. Little by little, as those changes are repeated over time the individual learns how to self-control his or her changed environment.

Vocational Training Programs in Asake Gakuen

We believe that a major goal for autistic adolescents and adults (as for normal adults) is to facilitate social independence. However, most autistic adults are also mentally retarded and typically maintain some autistic behaviors. In this section, we summarize our training program to help them achieve as much social independence as is possible.

Managing Vocational Task Situations

All of our residents work from Monday to Friday and at least 4 hours a day (Table 6). To manage a vocational task situation, the essence is that the vocational program be structured, with a schedule for all times during the day. (In contrast, the residential situation has a homey atmosphere.) Thus vocational units should be separated from residential units.

Table 7 shows the job environments and skills required in Asake Gakuen. We have incorporated many of the community's industries, so our residents can be adequately evaluated by the people of the community. Of course the on-site work and external workshop are outside our facilities. Some of the residents can eventually move from a sheltered (internal) workshop to an external workshop an on-site work. The external workshop is at a neighboring factory, where various occupations are undertaken. Every morning the residents who are able go to work on their bicycles.

Vocational skills and behaviors are important when undertaking job placements. It was found that vocational skills were related to motor skills and the requirements of

Table 7. Job environments in Asake Gakuen.

Department	Situation	Posture	Motor skills	Job responsibilities
On-site work	External/various	Various	Various	Various
External workshop	External/indoor	Sitting	Fingers and hand	Nut-and-bolt assembly, matching parts
Woodwork	Internal/indoor	Standing	Hand and arm	Polishing coasters, etc.
Farm and garden	Internal/outdoor	Locating	Gross motor	Growing vegetables

the job, and that vocational behaviors were related to the residents' postures. In our programs, maintained postures followed the completion of many adaptive behaviors (e.g., tense–relax muscles, assist with another hand, and eye–hand coordination). Furthermore, it is evident that maintaining a posture increased the task endurance. The goal of internal workshops is to master appropriate behaviors. There are two departments (woodworking and farming) with different levels of motor and cognitive skills.

Comprehension of Reward (Payment)

To facilitate social independence, it is neccessary to establish a vocational-residential training program that takes into account the difficulties autistic individuals have relating to others because of their language-cognitive disorders. Work is thus a medium for social learning. We have developed a strategy (working—comprehension of reward—profit) for daily life (Fig. 1): (1) promote the idea that one must work during one's lifetime. (2) recognize that job evaluation is equal to social evaluation. In this model, comprehension of reward (payment) plays a significant role.

Figure 2 demonstrates the training program utilized for nut-and-bolt assembly in our external workshop. Initially, a worker is given a baseline (four kinds of counterboard), standardized 100-yen payment daily. When he has finished the assembly of his counterboard, he can stamp in his card. As a result of this exercise he learns

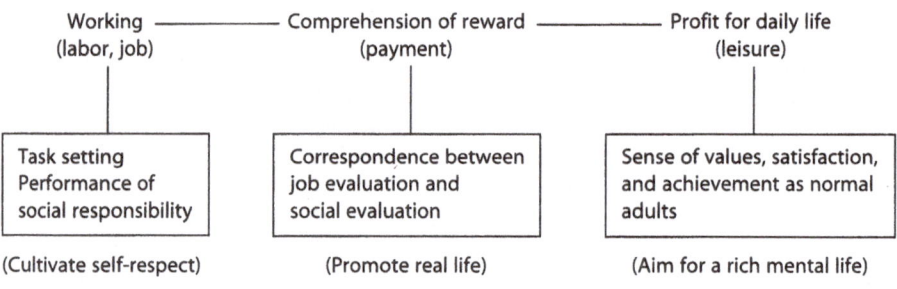

Fig. 1. Model for vocational-residential training program.

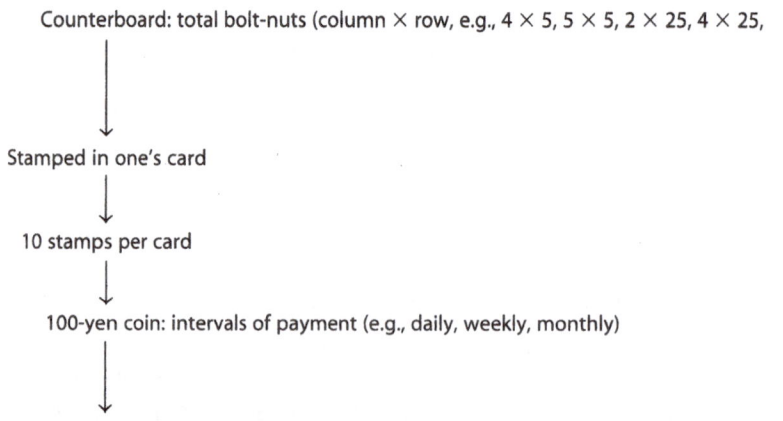

Fig. 2. Training program for comprehension of reward (payment).

the process by which a card stamped 10 times can be exchanged for a 100-yen coin. We have two interval schedules of payment: daily and weekly. Workers who have participated in this process for more than 12 months understand these rules and relate them to their ordinary needs. Characteristically, however, there are some who understand the rules but lack the desire to work voluntarily.

On-Site Work

After completing the training program that achieves comprehension of reward, the next goal is on-site work. Seven autistic adults are currently engaged in such work in our community. The intention of on-site work was originally to take another step toward regular employment. We have extended this application and apply it even to the more severely handicapped individuals. The records of three such autistic adults are outlined in Table 8.

Subjects of the Facility for Autistic Adults

The National Society for Autistic Children in Japan has reported that autistic disorders are considered a variety of developmental disabilities, so these individuals have been provided the same services offered the mentally retarded. A typical institution for autistic children was established in 1980. Moreover, most of the facilities for autistic adults are governed by the same policies used in those for the mentally retarded. However, autistic individuals require the continued operational expenses and therapeutic methodology into adulthood. The following problems exist in this field.

Placement of Staff

Direct-care staff members are limited to one per every 4.3 residents by statutory provision. At the facilities for autistic adults, the numbers are one per every 1.8 to 4.1 residents. It is a problem to have too few staff to administer the therapeutic program. If we did employ such staff we would have to do so according to these proportions.

It must be emphasized that the staff of a general institution has a prearranged management approach established for the overall facilities. Their duties can hardly deal with individuals who are severely autistic. Some of the facilities for autistic adults have a program in which the residents can go home every weekend, as enough staffs

Table 8. Autistic patients ($n = 3$) with on-site work.

Parameter	J.I.	M.S.	C.M.
Sex	Male	Male	Female
Age (years/months)	21/3	22/2	21/0
Binet's IQ (years/months)	15/9	8/2	14/8
Vineland's SA (years/months)	9/0	8/3	6/3
Period (years)	4.5	4.5	2.5
Job	Pottery	Pottery	Making cakes
Working hours (per week)	44	44	44
Transportation	Bicycle	Bicycle	Bus and train

cannot be maintained for those days. Because of the progressive individualistic approach for autistic people, for every 40 residents we need a clinical psychologist, occupational therapist, speech therapist, psychiatric social worker, recreation worker (coordinating music, sport, and art therapy), doctor, and two nurses.

Structure of Therapeutic Units

Each facilities for autistic adults houses a different variety of residents, from all autistic persons to those with four levels of retardation (profound, severe, moderate, mild) and other impairments. According to these structural differences, we must incorporate various policies that cover the particular facility and local situation.

The individuals who had received adequate psychiatric treatment previously can maintain some human relationships and so require only minimum staffs. In contrast, those whose prior treatment was insufficient require more hospitable management and hence more staff members. We propose that facilities for autistic adults should be organized based on the therapeutic principles used in the institution for autistic children.

Policy for Care of the Autistic Adult

Facilities for autistic adults should meet a number of needs, including short-term training, residential care, and emergency residence. Unfortunately, few facilities offer a program to helpless adults living at home. In this regard we have failed to design a policy for a therapeutic approach that meets the needs of individuals with an autistic disorder or to make use of case conferences, observational records, or psychiatric consultations.

Parents–Autistic Person Relationships

The relationship between parents and autistic residents and the facilities' staffs is currently being worked out on a trial-and-error basis. Particularly when the parents had something to do with the establishment of the facilities, some sentiment and acting-out as an owner or egoist tends to intervene in the guidance situation. In such cases the relationships between parents and staff members requires additional efforts.

Parental interventions are based on four factors.

1. Because the exact nature of autistic disorders have not been well described in the educational and welfare areas, parents seldom take advice regarding their children's upbringing. They only reluctantly have personally tackled many of the problems of their children.
2. Consequently, in facilities promoted and organized by a group of parents, there is a risk of exceeding the parents' authority in terms of management.
3. The parents often exhibit some distorted behaviors (e.g., replacement and reaction formation) owing to an unconscious feeling of guilt for having "abandoned" their beloved children to the facilities.
4. The parents want to feel secure that the care of their children will be assured after their death.

Conclusion

The care of autistic children and adults is incorporated into the treatment system for the mentally retarded in Japan. Although facilities for autistic children has been in existence, those for autistic adolescents and adults still have to be established under the current social system. Perhaps it is because of the view that it is difficult to distinguish autism from mental retardation in adults.

In actuality, many autistic adults are still maladjusted and residing in rehabilitation institutions for the mentally retarded, are incarcerated in psychiatric hospitals, or are having a miserable existence at home. Against this background parents of autistic people have organized facilities for them, Asake Gakuen. We have described this facilities for autistic adults. Finally, the Association for Facilities for Autistic Adults was established in 1987 and aims to accelerate a movement to realize the building of advanced facilities for autistic adults.

Bibliography

Cohen DJ, Donnellan AM (1987) Handbook of autism and pervasive developmental disorders. Wiley, New York, pp 384–395

Stokes K (1977) Planning for the future of a severely handicapped autistic child. J Autism Child Schizoph 7:288–298

Sullivan R (1977) Parents speak: needs of the older child, introduction. J Autism Child Schizoph 7:287–288

Psychosexual Development of Autistic Children During Adolescence

Ryuji Kobayashi

Summary. In the clinical field of autism, puberty or adolescence is a critical period. The psychosexual development of autistic children during adolescence was investigated, especially from the viewpoint of establishing gender identity formation. Some problems are proposed: the difficulty of establishing gender role identity during preadolescence, control of the growing sexual drive, perverse behavior, obsessiveness about body image, and the difficulty of establishing a relationship with a sexual partner. Psychosexual development is thought to be facilitated through the influence of interpersonal relationships. Hence it is a difficult task for autistic children to establish gender identity.

Key words. Adolescence—Autism—Gender identity—Psychosexual development

During the course of psychological development puberty or adolescence is a critical period. It is especially so in autistic children because of their specific cognitive deficits and communicative handicaps [1–3]. Prime developmental tasks during adolescence are (1) knowing how to deal with the powerful sexual drive and (2) the establishment of relationships with peers or opposite-sex persons as a result of separation from their parents. The purpose here is to investigate the psychosexual development of the autistic child during adolescence through particular cases, especially from the viewpoint of their establishing gender identity [4]. Gender identity is discussed in the context of Tyson's theory [5]: core gender identity, gender role identity, and sexual partner orientation.

Case Reports

The following eight case studies demonstrate the sexual problems of autistic children during adolescence.

Difficulty of Gender Role Identity

Case 1

This 11-year-old boy has an IQ of 106 (Tanaka-Binet). He tends to speak and behave as a girl.

Tokai University School of Health Sciences, Bohseidai, Isehara, Kanagwa 259-11, Japan

Fig. 1. Girl drawn by patient 1.
Fig. 2. Boy drawn by patient 1.

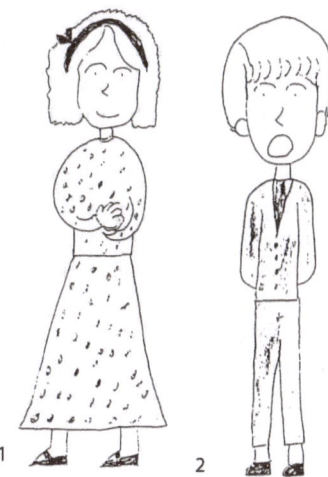

1   2

In early infancy he exhibited gaze aversion, hyperkinesis, and restlessness. When he was 2 years of age he stopped speaking and was diagnosed as autistic. When he was 3 years of age he resumed speaking but only with echolalic speech for the next few years. His father gave him speech training using a behavior modification technique, so enthusiastically that the boy came to feel intimidated by men. In kindergarten, he could not separate himself from his mother. After he entered a normal class in elementary school, his ability to speak progressed steadily, but he played only with female classmates. He came to speak and behave in the same manner as his female friends. He enjoyed learning knitting from his mother and was occupied with playing the piano. He pretended to have female breasts like his female classmates, putting a ball of paper in his shirt. He tied his hair with a hairband. He would hike up his shorts, pretending to be wearing high-cut women's swimwear. He was not ashamed at all of such behavior. He was sensitive, however, to the assessment of his school performance. When asked to draw a person, he drew a girl (Fig. 1). He was then asked to draw a boy and drew the picture shown in Figure 2. These pictures displayed his feminine tendencies. When he was 12 years of age, he said, "Keep this a secret between you and me: I was told not to use a feminine word. If I use it, I will be bullied by a classmate. So I will try not to use such words." Gradually, he tried to modify his own behavior.

Problems Concerning Control of the Growing Sexual Drive

Case 2

This 13-year-old boy has a TIQ of 61 (VIQ 47, PIQ 84) (WISC-R). He shouts at his mother loudly and frequently acts out behavior symbolic of masturbation.

When he was 1.5 years of age, he became hyperkinetic. He was preoccupied with manipulating machine toys. He enjoyed memorizing the names of Shinkansen (Super-Express) Line stations. He was enrolled in a special class in elementary school. When he was 9.5 years of age motor and vocal tics appeared and developed. He was diagnosed as suffering from Tourette's syndrome. When 11 years of age, he began to speak in a rough, aggressive manner. He had heard pupils in his school speak roughly, and he wanted to imitate their language. He criticized his mother's language in detail.

He said, "You should talk like this, not the way you do. It is not right." He was obsessed with her language. He imitated a favorite television detective and grew excited while speaking. He disobeyed his mother vehemently but at the same time was dependent on her. He wanted to cook with her, clinging to her and touching her breasts.

When he was 13 years of age he was ashamed to look when his sister changed her clothes, although he was willing to watch his mother change without shame, often saying, "I am watching you." Rough language was escalated. He used obscene slang without hesitation or sense of taboo. He would harshly tell his mother to leave, but if she actually started to leave he would stop her at the porch, begging earnestly, "Please don't leave." His sexual drive increased. At one point he took a sausage from the refrigerator, grasping it with both hands over tissue paper. This behavior symbolized masturbation. Even now he is sometimes preoccupied with such behavior, but he is adapting well socially.

Case 3

A 15-year-old boy with an IQ of 40 and his mother are anxious about mutual separation prior to his entering a boarding school. When he was 2 years of age, he was diagnosed as autistic. Both he and his mother have had anxiety about separation, and his mother brought him up rather obsessively. Even when he was a student in junior high school, she kept him under strict observation. One day, he was found masturbating in his bed and was scolded by her. After that, he began to masturbate while saying, "Don't do this! Don't do this!" He was fond of watching a certain television news program and especially liked a particular female newscaster. However, when she was speaking, he turned down the volume. When the male newscaster began to speak, he turned the volume to its original level, thereby denying his feelings for the opposite sex. He was suffering from guilt feelings after the masturbation incident with his mother.

Problems of Intensified Curiosity about Heterosexuality

Case 4

A 13-year-old boy with VIQ undetermined and a PIQ of 66 (WISC-R), is restless, exhibits questionmania (klagesuchtig), and is maladapted at school. He is an only child. His father works excessively and is rarely present, so mother and child are living essentially alone. His mother is unstable and lacked confidence in bringing him up. When he was in a upper grade in elementary school, he could not achieve a satisfactory performance and was maladaptive and isolated. He became obsessive.

In junior high school, he began to behave problematically. He has been in normal classes even in junior high school, but he has not been able to make friends and is isolated. He peeped into the girls' locker room, approached a girl inappropriately, and tripped one girl intentionally. He showed strong curiosity about heterosexuality. It is suggested that when his curiosity about heterosexuality became overwhelming he began to act in this direct manner.

Case 5

A 21-year-old man with TIQ undetermined (VIQ undetermined, PIQ 76) (WAIS) has problematical behavior toward girls and women. He is an only child, and when he was

4 years of age he was diagnosed as being autistic. When a toddler, he was phobic about anything with a round shape. He was clumsy yet was talented in limited areas. When he entered junior college, he began to live separately from his mother for the first time, where he had always been under her strict control. She used to tell him. "Don't do what you don't like to be done." In this, he was obedient to his mother. When he was at the boarding house, the manageress let him see a magazine with nude photographs. He became upset and told her not to look at such magazines. When he saw a young female student on the street, he quickly averted his eyes from her. He denied his interest in females, but it was revealed that he was displaying problematic behavior toward them. He intentionally touched some female students, threatened them, or suddenly gave them an unprovoked kick. His behavior was seriously problematical, but he was fortunately able to graduate from college and get a job. He is now adapting to the job.

Problems of Perverse Behavior

Case 6

An 18-year-old young man with an IQ of 59 has an elder sister and a younger brother. He is fair colored and good-looking. When he was 4 years of age, he was diagnosed as autistic. At age 12 years he began to suffer from epilepsy. At that time his father went fishing with him, but they never spoke to each other. His brother criticized him for his unusual behavior. When he was 16 years old, he began to pull out his pubic hair and in an orderly fashion lay it on the toilet seat. He stole his sister's swimsuit and took baths while wearing it. He was believed to have also taken it to his room to wear. He was left to do as he wished. He collected erotic articles from sports newspapers. He covered the television screen when a slim girl appeared on it wearing tight jeans. When his family told him he was being obscene, he would smirk. He showed strong curiosity about heterosexuality. He said directly say to his mother, "I want to touch your breasts and legs. I want to lick you."

He could not urinate in a standing position; he urinated in a sitting position. He could not unzip his trousers to urinate. He was obsessive about cleanliness and as an infant could not hold an onigiri (rice ball) directly with his fingers. Nor could he directly touch his penis with his fingers.

Problems Regarding the Diffusion of Body Image

Case 7

A 23-year-old woman with an IQ of 45 displays obsessiveness and a strong inferiority complex about her figure. When she was 4 years old she was diagnosed as autistic. When she was 8 years old she developed a strong sense of curiosity about her personal appearance and makeup. Her drawing (Fig. 3) demonstrates her strong sense of curiosity. When she was in the second year of high school, the breasts of her only friend began to develop. The patient was so obsessed by this development that she began to peep inside her friend's dress. From that point, she grew obsessive about her figure and body image. She could not look straight at another person, averting her eyes. She believed that her mother, brother, and many others had beautiful hair and figures. As for her own appearance, she believed she looked strange and ugly. She said that since infancy her hair, face, and mind all had seemed strange. During this time

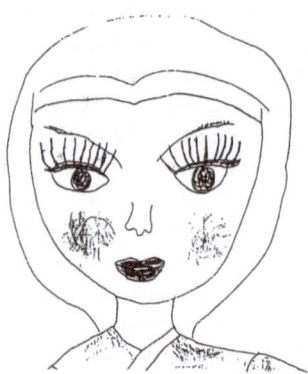

Fig. 3. Girl drawn by patient 7.

she was unable to look straight not only at people but also at some female figures. Even the image of a fish on a chopping board frightened her. She became afraid of looking at such pictures and covered them with her hand. In an early interview, it became clear that her mother had been a compulsive dieter and had had some conflict with the formation of gender identity in her youth. At the time the patient became shocked by her friend's breast development, her father had been suffering from cancer, which soon resulted in his death. Therefore her mother could not show any concern for her daughter's anxiety at that time.

Problems of the Need for Heterosexual Live Objects

Case 8

A 16-year-old girl [TIQ 80 (VIQ 84, PIQ 79) (WISC-R)] lost her self-esteem and reacted with panic. She was extremely sensitive to her differences, and this sensitivity intensified the panic. She was an only child. There were no problems during the prenatal period, and birth and physical development were normal. As an infant she had a poor response to her mother and no anxiety toward strangers. A dependency on her mother was not noticeable. Her speech was delayed. She did not utter any words that were understandable until she was 3 years old. At age 3 she became hyperkinetic and was so sensitive to certain sounds, such as a baby's cry, that she sometimes reacted violently. At age 4 she started kindergarten, but she could not behave socially as the other children did. She was referred to a child guidance clinic and diagnosed as autistic. At home she was preoccupied with putting whisky bottles in a straight line and writing and drawing on the walls.

When she entered elementary school, she was placed in normal classes. She occupied her time by consulting the Kanji character dictionary every day. She learned so many Kanji characters that she was called the "Queen of Kanji characters" by her classmates. In the fifth grade (elementary school), she was referred to a child guidance clinic because of restlessness, hyperkinesis, and violent behavior in school. She had special skills in writing many Kanji characters but poor skills in calculating and reading. She was advised to go to a special class for the mentally handicapped. However, she entered junior high school and was placed in normal classes. In the seventh grade (junior high school), she became too restless to stay in her classroom for even an hour. Gradually she began to wonder who she was. In the ninth grade she became aware that she was suffering from autism. She realized that she could not do things as well as the other pupils could. Even after she realized that she was different from the other classmates, her behavior did not change. Instead she became compulsive about smelling her classmates' hair.

After graduating from junior high school, she entered a special technical school for dressmaking near her home. At that time, her behavior changed. She became friendly to her classmates, became more emotionally stable, and showed more interest in being properly dressed. She became so independent that she started to go to school by herself. She became absorbed in learning how to make dresses, but she behaved inappropriately so often that her classmates criticized her for her odd behavior. She became sensitive to being criticized and so sensitive about her self-esteem that it escalated into a state of panic. Soon after that, she was referred to my clinic. She was given pimozide 1–2 mg/day, which resulted in her becoming calm. Her intelligence was tested as TIQ 80 (VIQ 84, PIQ 79) by WISC-R.

九州電力

Fig. 4. Kanji characters of Kyu-Shu-Den-Ryoku.

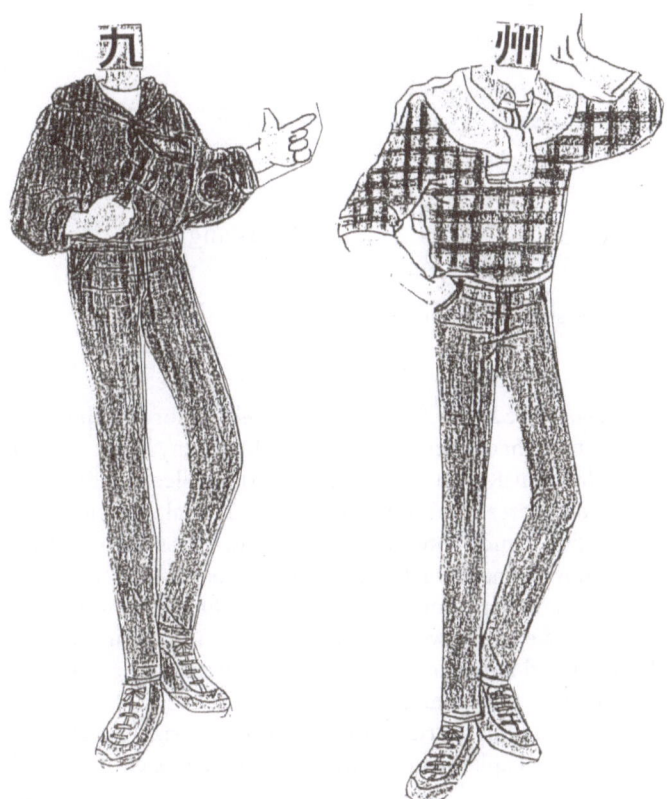

Fig. 5. Kyu-kun and Shu-kun.

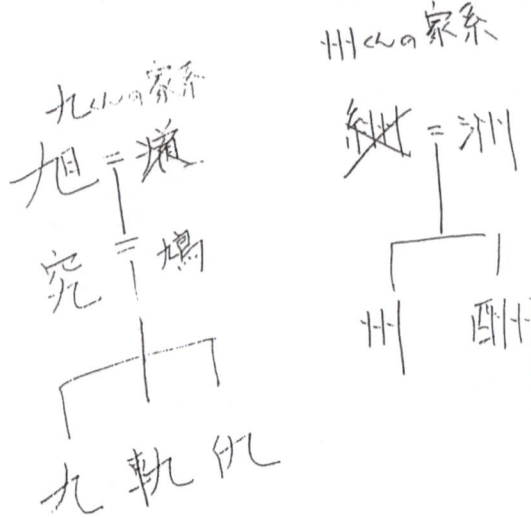

Fig. 6. Genograms for Kyu-kun and Shu-kun.

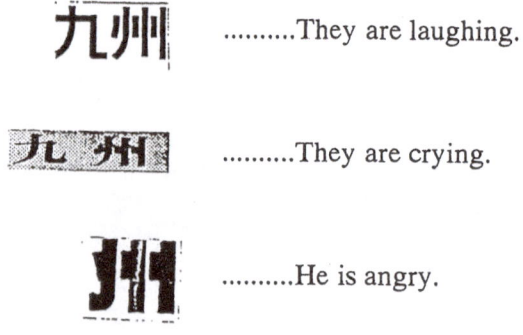

Fig. 7. Some emotional states of Kyu-kun and Shu-kun.

During adolescence she began to have strong feelings for members of the opposite sex. Because of that, she had a strong desire to collect many kinds of Kanji characters, specifically Kyu-Shu-Den-Ryoku (meaning the Kyushu Electronic Company) (Fig. 4). Each Kanji character represented to her an imaginary male classmate (Fig. 5), so she called them, "Kyu-kun"[1] and "Shu-kun." She imagined them as boyfriends. When she was alone, she enjoyed speaking to them in her room. She collected these Kanji characters from the newspaper and kept them under her pillow while sleeping. In the morning when she woke up she would say, "Good morning, Kyu-kun. Good morning, Shu-kun." She described Kyu-kun as being talented in sports, belonging to the basketball club, and being the president of the high school. As for Shu-kun, she described him also as being talented in sports and very smart. Surprisingly, she also made their genograms (Fig. 6). She explained that the Kanji characters each had emotions, such

---

[1] In Japanese, "*Kun*" is a term added to the end of a proper name to show friendship or fondness for the person being mentioned. It functions the same as "*San*," which is the formal Japanese for Mr./Ms.

as "They are angry", "They are crying" "They are laughing" (Fig. 7). To her their emotions seemed different according to the typeface style of the characters. Although she was enthusiastic about collecting Kanji characters and imagining Kanji characters as real people, her daily life activities were based in reality, receiving some advice from her teachers and me.

Discussion

How do autistic adolescents establish gender identity? Having discussed these problems through the case reports, I now propose some points.

The first is the problem of the diffusion of establishing gender role identity. As case 1 indicates, some autistic adolescents are so apt to avoid same-sex friendships because of phobia about boys that they introject the behavior of girls superficially. Others introject the aggressive behavior of boys too dogmatically.

The second is the problem of confusion caused by an ambivalence between the heightened sexual drive and the dependency needs on the mother. Mothers who have preadolescent autistic children are apt to be so perplexed or confused that they tend to approach the children too closely and with excessive concern. If children's behavior is too strictly criticized, they then develop guilt feelings about masturbation.

The third point is the problem that intensified curiosity about heterosexuality sometimes causes an uncontrollable sexual drive. The masturbation stage of curiosity is dealt with in the family. However, when the curiosity about heterosexuality is heightened to an uncontrollable degree, it causes difficulties. Such difficulties may be related to the cognitive deficit and confusion regarding the differences of heterosexuality.

The fourth problem is that of perverse behaviors. This problem is not recognized until the therapeutic relationship has deepened. To satisfy their sexual drive, some autistic adolescents touch, wear, or smell their mothers' or sisters' shorts or clothes.

The fifth problem is specific to females regarding the diffusion of the body image. The somatic spurt during adolescence brings about confusion of body image, and it provides an opportunity to form a new body image. Autistic adolescents, however, who have difficulty differentiating self and others, are apt to be obsessive about the differences of others in detail. It is difficult for them to alleviate their psychopathology.

The last problem is concerned with the needs for heterosexual love objects. It is the most difficult problem for an autistic adolescent. It is natural that they have longings for heterosexual persons. They are apt to be enthusiastic about singing idols, for example, but they tend to avoid actual relationships with opposite-sex persons, so it is difficult to make a change from simple longing to a true heterosexual relationship. This point is illustrated in case 8, where the Kanji characters have recently begun to be perceived by the patient not as inanimate things but as real persons. Each is described by her to have a brilliant career and she has provided detailed genograms. During adolescence she began to display a strong sense of self-consciousness and strong feelings for members of the opposite sex. Her strong feelings for male persons and her strong desire to collect many kinds of Kanji characters are probably interrelated. Her strong feelings might make it possible to perceive the Kanji characters as real persons, or "physiognomically" [6].

Above all, it is true that autistic adolescents have mental characteristics specific to adolescence according to their chronological age. Psychosexual development in humans should be achieved through the influence of human relationships. Anxiety about sex may be lessened in these relationships and is integrated into the ego. For autistic adolescents, however, who have core difficulties with relationships, it may be a severe developmental task to obtain a sexual partner.

References

1. Gillberg C, Schaumann H (1989) Autism: specific problems of adolescence. In: Gillberg C (ed) Diagnosis and treatment of autism. Plenum, New York, 375
2. Kobayashi R, Murata T (1990) Qu'est-ce qui est important pour que des autistes deviennent à l'âge adulte indépendants ou capables de subvenir à leurs besoins? In: Chiland C, Young JG (eds) Nouvelles approches de la santé mentale: de la naissance à l'adolescence pour l'enfant et sa famille. Presses Universitaires de France, Paris, pp 333–346
3. Schopler E, Mesibov G (eds) (1983) Autism in adolescents and adults. Plenum, New York
4. Stoller RJ (1968) Sex and gender. Science House, New York
5. Tyson P (1982) A developmental line of gender identity, gender role and choice of love object. J Am Psychoanal Assoc 30:61–86
6. Werner H (1948) Comparative psychology of mental development. Follett, Chicago

Regression in Mental Development Following a Psychosocial Stressor in Disintegrative Psychosis

Hiroshi Kurita,[1] Takamasa Saito,[1] and Michiko Kita[2]

Summary. A psychosocial stressor preceding mental regression was studied in 22 patients with disintegrative psychosis (DP) and compared with 58 patients with infantile autism (IA) with speech loss. It was significantly more common in the 22 DP patients (63.6%) than in the 58 IA patients (34.5%). Finger-pointing existed before regression significantly more often in 14 DP patients with a psychosocial stressor (71.4%) than the other 8 patients without it (12.5%), whereas head circumference at birth was significantly smaller in 13 (mean 33.0 cm) of the former than in 6 (mean 34.8 cm) of the latter. The 14 DP patients appear to have developed sufficiently to be able to react psychologically against a stressor. Such a reaction might trigger regression depending on the vulnerability of the brain.

Key words. Childhood disintegrative disorder—Disintegrative psychosis—Infantile autism

Regression of mental development sometimes occurs during infancy. Its manifestations vary from temporary psychological regression in a sibling of a newborn baby to fatal regression in a child with a neurodegenerative disease. Between these two extremes there exists a largely irreversible yet not lethal type of regression. Such a regression has been reported most frequently with pervasive developmental disorders (PDDs) [1–6].

Mental regression has become not only an important research theme but also a key feature when classifying some varieties of PDD. It has been suggested to distinguish infantile autism that shows regression in speech development as its subtype [3, 4]. The ICD-10 classification [7] introduced two new categories (i.e., Rett Syndrome and Other Childhood Disintegrative Disorder), both characterized by regression in mental development, in the class of PDD. Both were adopted in the final draft of the *Diagnostic and Statistical Manual, 4th Edition (DSM-IV)* [8].

Regression of mental development in PDD requires more study. One area for such study is the role of a psychosocial stressor preceding regression in some PDD cases. Because such a stressor is not rare during early infancy and tends to be recalled by

---

[1] Department of Mental Health, Faculty of Medicine, University of Tokyo, 7-3-1 Hongo, Bunkyo-ku, Tokyo 113, Japan
[2] National Institute of Mental Health, NCNP, 1-7-3 Konodai, Ichikawa, Chiba 272, Japan

parents as it relates to the regression, many authors [6, 9–12] have not considered it causally important in mental regression.

However, among cases of dementia infantilis [13] or Heller's syndrome (or its modern name, disintegrative psychosis) [14], which presents a clear mental regression after normal or near-normal development, there are those who appear to have regressed after a psychosocial stressor. Four of Heller's [13] six patients with dementia infantilis had had psychosocial stressors (i.e., hospital admission for resection of adenoids, moving, fear of dogs, and falling from a car without injury) before regression. Of 10 disintegrative psychosis patients reported by Evans-Jones and Rosenbloom [2], six had had psychosocial stressors before their mental disintegration.

Psychosocial stressors preceding regression in other representative cases of disintegrative psychosis (or by whatever other name it may be called) were (1) the father's entering the army—a boy with Heller's syndrome [15]; (2) an air raid during World War II—a boy with dementia infantilis [16]; (3) sexual assault—a girl with Heller's dementia [17]; (4) a parental quarrel—a boy with Heller's syndrome [18]; (5) moving—a girl with Heller's dementia [19]; (6) a strenuous automobile trip—a boy with dementia infantilis [20]; and (7) birth of a sibling—a boy with disintegrative psychosis [21]. In some autism cases a psychosocial stressor also appears to have triggered the manifestation of autistic symptoms [4, 22].

Although the combination of a psychosocial stressor and vulnerability of the brain seems important in the causation of mental regression, a data-based study to address this point is still lacking. In this study, we tried to clarify the role and characteristics of a psychosocial stressor in mental regression of disintegrative psychosis, where such regression seems most clearly presented, based on the largest sample ever reported.

Method

Subjects

To diagnose cases of disintegrative psychosis (DP), we used the ICD-9 [14] definition of DP. Because the lower limit of the age of onset was unclear in this definition, we set it at 2 years, as was proposed in the ICD-10 draft's [23] diagnostic criteria for other childhood disintegrative disorders.

We selected DP patients consecutively among referrals to two facilities well known in Tokyo for specializing in the developmentally disabled: the Nerima Welfare Center for the Mentally and Physically Handicapped and the Child Guidance Center affiliated with the National Welfare Foundation for Disabled Children from 1980 to 1992. We included only DP patients under age 16 at their first visit, as we had done in a previous study [5]. Detailed clinical examinations of children in both facilities are described elsewhere [4, 5].

Twenty-two children (mean age ± SD 6.5 ± 2.5 years; 17 boys, 5 girls) were diagnosed as having DP by two of us (H.K. and M.K.), both child psychiatrists, based on chart review. H.K. examined and followed up 21 of the 22 DP patients. Of the 22 DP patients, 20 (90.9%) had mental retardation of moderate grade or below. The mean age at onset of regression was 2.7 ± 0.6 years. Of the 22 DP patients; 9 also met the ICD-10 draft criteria for Other Childhood Disintegrative Disorder (OCDD).

As a contrast group, we selected 58 consecutive patients with infantile autism (IA) who showed similar regression (i.e., IA with speech loss) under age 16 at first visit (age

6.1 ± 3.3 years; 44 boys; 14 girls) to the same two facilities during the same time as the DP patients. They all satisfied *DSM-III* [24] diagnostic criteria for IA. Based on a clinical record of language development noted by a speech pathologist or psychologist, we confirmed that the 58 IA patients had shown speech loss, defined by Kurita [4] and summarized as follows: (1) an episode wherein the child lost all meaningful words expressed spontaneously in a situation, such as requesting food; and (2) after the disappearance of speech, the child remained mute for at least 6 months.

Procedure

A psychosocial stressor was identified from detailed descriptions of a child's early development by psychologists based on interviews with parents. The severity and type (acute or enduring) of a psychosocial stressor were evaluated on the *DSM-III-R* [25] scale.

We rated levels of mental development of children before regression on a 2-point scale in three areas: speech ("phrases or sentences" and "single words only"); interpersonal–social relationships ("normal" and "not entirely normal"); and fingerpointing ("presence" and "absence").

The comparison was made in two steps. First, we compared the incidence of a psychosocial stressor before regression between the DP patients and IA patients with speech loss. Next, we compared the DP patients with and without a psychosocial stressor before regression regarding variables that preceded the regression, including prenatal and birth histories, developmental landmarks, and the levels of mental development before regression.

Results

Incidence and Characteristics of Psychosocial Stressors

Of the 22 DP patients, 14 (63.6%) had had a psychosocial stressor before regression, whereas 20 (34.5%) of the 58 IA patients with speech loss did; there was a significant difference between them: χ^2 ($n = 80$) = 5.55; $P < 0.05$. The incidence of a psychosocial stressor before regression, however, did not differ significantly between the 9 OCDD (66.7%) patients and the other 13 non-OCDD DP (61.5%) patients.

The severity of a psychosocial stressor on the *DSM-III-R* scale did not differ significantly between the 14 DP patients (mean ± SD 2.5 ± 0.7) and the 20 IA patients with speech loss (2.5 ± 0.6). The type of psychosocial stressor was "acute" in all 14 DP and 20 IA patients. Only four DP patients and one IA patient had multiple stressors.

Patients With and Without Psychosocial Stressors

The head circumference at birth was significantly smaller in 13 of the 14 DP patients with a psychosocial stressor (mean ± SD 33.0 ± 1.6 cm) than in 6 of the 8 DP patients without it (34.8 ± 1.1 cm), [t(17) = 2.46; $P < 0.05$], whereas body weight, body length, and chest circumference at birth did not differ significantly between the two DP groups. The two DP groups did not differ significantly in terms of gestational age, maternal age at delivery, the incidence of an individual obstetrical risk factor, and mean number of risk factors in an infant. They also did not differ significantly in terms of initial age at head control, sitting, walking, and speaking.

The rate of patients having developed finger-pointing before regression was significantly higher in the 14 DP patients with a psychosocial stressor (10 cases, 71.4%) than in the other 8 without it (1 case, 12.5%) (Fisher's test, $P < 0.05$). The rate did not differ significantly between speech loss IA patients with and without a psychosocial stressor before speech loss. It also did not differ significantly between the 13 non-OCDD DP patients (38.5%) and 9 OCDD cases (66.7%).

Of the 14 DP patients with a psychosocial stressor before regression, 6 (42.9%) and 11 (78.6%) had a two-word phrase or sentence and normal interpersonal–social relationships before regression, respectively. However, the levels of speech and interpersonal–social relationships before regression did not differ significantly between DP patients with and without a psychosocial stressor before regression.

Case Reports

Case 1

A boy with OCDD was aged 9 years 8 months at the time of his first examination (by H.K.). The natal period was uneventful. He was a product of his mother's first pregnancy and weighed 3270 g. Although a forceps was used at delivery, he had no asphyxia and had icterus of normal grade. He passed early motor landmarks without delay and responded well to his parents. Before age 1 year he showed distress whenever his mother left him, and he crawled to follow her. At around age 1 he began to show a stranger anxiety. He liked his parents to do a peek-a-boo for him and tried to imitate it himself.

He uttered his initial speech at 11 months of age. He used pointing by finger before age 1.5 years. At the time of his health checkup at age 1.5 years, no abnormality was found by a pediatrician or a psychologist, as he had several meaningful words, finger-pointing, and good responsiveness to others. After that point his vocabulary expanded further. He tried to console his baby brother, 1.3 years younger than he, by offering him a toy whenever the baby cried.

After age 2.4 years a chain of misfortunes struck him. During the winter his parents were preparing for moving. Although he became anxious on seeing snowfall, he looked otherwise normal. A photograph taken before the move showed that the boy was helping his father pack by handing a nail to him. Just after the move he still looked normal. His parents remembered that he imitated actions of Japanese samurai on television programs.

Shortly after the move, at age 2.4 years, his second younger brother was born. Soon afterward, his maternal grandfather, to whom this boy had strongly attached, died. He then became anxious and fearful about falling snow. He gradually lost meaningful words as well as vivid and happy facial expressions. He liked to sit in the corner of the room at home with a vacant face. He was no longer joyful when going out with his family. He did not approach even his mother. He disliked parental interactions with him. He lost eye-to-eye contact. He began to look sideways and to exhibit hand-flapping. He lost bladder control, which had been established before the move. He started walking on tiptoe and then gradually showed a clumsy gait and reluctance to walk. However, his parents' efforts to help him walk enabled him to walk again: first, tiptoe walking and then normal walking. He persisted in holding a pillow. He liked to watch a rotating fan.

He remained in a regressed state for about 2 years after the onset of regression. However, at around age 6 years signs of recovery emerged. He started to use finger-pointing. He attained bladder and bowel control at age 6 years. At about the same time, he began to watch television, in which he had lost interest after regression.

At the initial examination by H.K. at age 9.7, he uttered few meaningful words. He became panicky on seeing a medical instrument in an examination room. He did not exhibit eye-to-eye contact, and he flapped his hands in front of his face. He stuck to licking and smelling things. His IQ was untestable, with the retardation level estimated as severe. The severity and type of his psychosocial stressors before regression were judged severe and acute on the *DSM-III-R* scale.

Clinical neurological examinations and an induced-sleep electroencephalogram disclosed no abnormality. He had mild dilatation of the sylvian fissure on a computed tomography (CT) scan.

A son of his mother's elder sister had speech retardation during infancy but got excellent school records later, though he is still clumsy and tends to persist in his routines. His family history showed no mood disorder.

Cases 2–14

As summarized in Table 1, all but one (no. 14) of the other 13 DP patients exhibited fearfulness as an early symptom before speech regression. Clinical charts of the 13 DP patients indicated that all of them had shown underresponsiveness to other persons along with speech regression and other autistic symptoms. There seems to be a possibility that most of the 13 DP patients reacted similarly to a psychosocial stressor.

Discussion

Given the limited number of cases, our results must be considered preliminary, though our DP sample is the largest one ever published. Another limitation of our study was that parental recollections were the sole informational source of a psychosocial stressor and mental regression. Thus a future study based on DP cases examined at much younger ages is needed. However, the basic features of our sample—mean age at onset of regression, male/female ratio, rate of moderate retardation or below, and rate of the appearance of a psychosocial stressor before regression (2.7 years, 3.4:1, 90.9%, and 63.6%, respectively)—did not differ significantly from the figures for the 10 DP patients in Evans-Jones and Rosenbloom's study (2.5 years, 4:1, 100%, and 60.0%, respectively) [2] and those for 10 cases of disintegrative disorder in Volkmar and Cohen's study (2.8 years, 10:0, 100%, and 70.0%, respectively) [6]. Therefore, the results of our study may be valid.

Histories of the 14 DP patients indicated that regression had occurred following a psychosocial stressor, as in many historical cases of DP [26]. Our finding that a psychosocial stressor preceded mental regression significantly more commonly in the DP cases than in IA cases with speech loss suggests that the DP patients had reacted to a psychosocial stressor more seriously than the IA patients with speech loss, given that there was no significant difference in the severity of a psychosocial stressor for the two conditions.

Table 1. Summary of 13 cases of disintegrative psychosis or other childhood disintegrative disorder with psychosocial stressor before regression.

Pt. no.	Sex	Dx[a]	Age of onset (year)	Psychosocial stressor	Severity[b] of psychosocial stressor	Early symptoms after psychosocial stressor and before speech regression
2	F	DP	4.5	Birth of sibling; enrolled in kindergarten	Moderate	Fearful; gloomy; stern face; agitated
3	M	DP	2.5	House repairs	Mild	Fearful; frequent crying
4	M	OCDD	2.1	Hospitalization	Mild	Fearful
5	M	DP	2.5	Birth of sibling	Moderate	Fearful; strongly jealous of a newborn brother
6	F	OCDD	2.7	Severe beating by father	Moderate	Fearful; lost smile; stiffened face
7	M	DP	2.5	Moving	Mild	Fearful; agitated during night
8	M	OCDD	2.0	Separation from grandmother	Mild	Fearful; crying for 3 days after grandmother's departure
9	M	DP	4.0	Enrollment in kindergarten	Mild	Fearful
10	M	OCDD	2.0	Hospitalization	Mild	Fearful
11	M	DP	3.0	Parental fight; moving	Moderate	Fearful; anxious about sounds
12	M	DP	3.0	Birth of sibling; not allowed to suck a handkerchief	Moderate	Fearful; sulky
13	F	OCDD	2.5	Bone fracture of the dominant left hand	Mild	Fearful; nervous; panicky
14	F	DP	3.0	Moving	Mild	No fearfulness

[a] Dx, diagnosis: DP, disintegrative psychosis in ICD-9; OCDD, Other Childhood Disintegrative Disorder in ICD-10.
[b] On the *DSM-III-R* scale. All psychosocial stressor types were acute.

An essential feature of the psychosocial stressors in the 14 DP cases seems to be a situation in which an infant is left by an attached person, object, or place. Such events make an infant depressed. In case 1 the patient developed a depressive state after a series of psychosocial stressors. Most of the other 13 patients seem to have reacted in an approximately similar fashion. Some historical cases of DP (or whatever it was called in the past) exhibited a similar state shortly after a psychosocial stressor and before regression. A boy with Heller's syndrome reported by Yakovlev et al. [15] became sad after his father entered the army and clung desperately to his mother whenever she left for her work place. These events occurred just before the onset of the boy's mental deterioration. A girl with Heller's dementia reported by Koupernik et al. [17] suffered from a nightmare and anxiety state before regression after sexual assault.

Psychosocial stressors such as those seen in our 14 patients are not necessarily rare during infancy. For example, young children facing the birth of a sibling sometimes show a psychological reaction, in which they are withdrawn or act like a baby. Such an event usually does not leave the child with a permanent problem. Why did our 14 DP patients regress beyond a benign reaction? As suggested in DP or OCDD patients [2, 5, 6], the 14 might already have had a vulnerability of the brain, even though it might have been milder in them than the other 8 DP patients.

A certain level of mental development is necessary for a child to perceive a psychosocial stressor as such and to display a psychological reaction, which could reduce the threshold of, or trigger, mental regression. This may be the reason why a psychosocial stressor was more important for regression in terms of speech loss in DP than IA patients. Our finding that the 14 DP patients with a psychosocial stressor before regression had significantly more advanced finger-pointing development before regression than the other 8 DP patients may confirm the need for fairly satisfactory development before regression. The mental development of the 14 DP patients with a psychosocial stressor before regression was more sufficient (allowing a psychological reaction to occur) than was the mental development of the 8 DP patients, but it was not sufficient to withstand the impact of the reaction that triggered regression.

A psychosocial stressor may not be as meaningful a factor for regression in IA patients with speech loss because its presence or absence was not significantly associated with the level of mental development before regression, as measured by the acquisition of finger-pointing in our autistic patients. IA with speech loss appears destined to regress regardless of whether a psychosocial stressor is present.

The DP patients who regressed after exposure to a psychosocial stressor appear to have attained seemingly normal, though precarious, mental development only to have it disturbed by a psychological reaction after the stressor appeared. Although our data indicating such precariousness or vulnerability were limited, the smaller head circumference at birth in the DP patients exposed to a psychosocial stressor before regression compared to the head circumference of those without a stressor might be a factor. Further studies based on early diagnosed cases of DP or OCDD are needed to clarify the mechanism of a psychosocial stressor that triggers regression as well as the vulnerability to mental regression in such cases.

In sum, regression after a psychosocial stressor was more common in DP patients than in IA patients with speech loss. DP patients with such an episode appear to have developed more sufficiently before regression than those without it, thereby being able to have a psychological reaction when facing a psychosocial stressor. Such a reaction might trigger mental regression, depending on the vulnerability of the brain.

Acknowledgments. This study was supported in part by Research Grant 5B-5-01 for Nervous and Mental Disorders from the Ministry of Health and Welfare, Japan. The authors thank Kaoru Katsuno in the Nerima Welfare Center for the Mentally and Physically Handicapped and Etsuko Yabe in the National Welfare Foundation for Disabled Children for their assistance in data collection.

References

1. Burd L, Fisher W, Kerbeshian J (1988) Childhood onset pervasive developmental disorder. J Child Psychol Psychiatry 29:155–163
2. Evans-Jones LG, Rosenbloom L (1978) Disintegrative psychosis in childhood. Dev Med Child Neurol 20:462–470
3. Hoshino Y, Kaneko M, Yashima Y, Kumashiro H, Volkmar FR, Cohen DJ (1987) Clinical features of autistic children with setback course in their infancy. Jpn J Psychiatr Neurol 41:237–246
4. Kurita H (1985) Infantile autism with speech loss before the age of thirty months. J Am Acad Child Psychiatry 24:191–196
5. Kurita H, Kita M, Miyake Y (1992) A comparative study of development and symptoms among disintegrative psychosis and infantile autism with and without speech loss. J Autism Dev Disord 22:175–188
6. Volkmar FR, Cohen DJ (1989) Disintegrative disorder or "late onset" autism. J Child Psychol Psychiatry 30:717–724
7. World Health Organization (1992) The ICD-10 classification of mental disorders: clinical descriptions and diagnostic guidelines. World Health Organization, Geneva
8. American Psychiatric Association (1993) DSM-IV draft criteria: 1/3/93. American Psychiatric Association, Washington, DC
9. Cantwell DP, Baker L, Rutter M (1978) Family factors. In: M Rutter, E Schopler (eds) Autism: a reappraisal of concepts and treatment. Plenum, New York, pp 269–296
10. Hill AE, Rosenbloom L (1986) Disintegrative psychosis of childhood: teenage follow-up. Dev Med Child Neurol 28:34–40
11. Rutter M (1968) Concepts of autism: a review of research. J Child Psychol Psychiatry 9:1–25
12. Rutter M (1985) Infantile autism and other pervasive developmental disorders. In: M Rutter, L Hersov (eds) Child and adolescent psychiatry: modern approaches, 2nd ed. Blackwell, Oxford, pp 545–566
13. Heller T (1908) Über Dementia infantilis: Verblödungsprozess im Kindesalter. Z Erforsch Behandl Jugendl Schwachsinns 2:17–28
14. World Health Organization (1977) International classification of diseases, 1975 revision, vol 1. World Health Organization, Geneva
15. Yakovlev PI, Weinberger M, Chipman CE (1948) Heller's syndrome as a pattern of schizophrenic behavior disturbance in early childhood. Am J Ment Defic 53:318–337
16. Hudolin V (1957) Dementia infantilis Heller: diagnostic problems with a case report. J Ment Defic Res 1:79–90
17. Koupernik C, Masciangelo PM, Balestra-Beretta S (1972) A case of Heller's dementia following sexual assault in a four-year-old girl. Child Psychiatry Hum Dev 2:134–144
18. Chmiel AJ, Mattson A (1975) Heller's syndrome: a form of childhood psychosis of multicausal origin. J Am Acad Child Psychiatry 14:337–347
19. Korey SR, Winograd H (1959) Biochemical alterations in a case of Heller's disease. Am J Dis Child 97:668–675
20. Roy I (1959) Zur Frage der Dementia infantilis Heller. Helv Paediatr Acta 14:288–301
21. Kurita H (1988) A case of Heller's syndrome with school refusal. J Autism Dev Disord 18:315–319
22. Burd L, Kerbeshian J (1988) Psychogenic and neurodevelopmental factors in autism. J Am Acad Child Adolesc Psychiatry 27:252–253
23. World Health Organization (1990) ICD-10. Chapter V: Mental and behavioural disorders (including disorders of psychological development): diagnostic criteria for research (May 1990 draft for field trials). World Health Organization, Geneva
24. American Psychiatric Association (1980) Diagnostic and statistical manual of mental disorders, 3rd ed. American Psychiatric Association, Washington, DC
25. American Psychiatric Association (1987) Diagnostic and statistical manual of mental disorders, 3rd ed revised. American Psychiatric Association, Washington, DC
26. Kurita H (1988) The concept and nosology of Heller's syndrome: review of articles and report of two cases. Jpn J Psychiatr Neurol 42:785–793

Longitudinal Study on Treatment and Outcome for Autistic Children

Masatsugu Hayashi, Issei Takamura, Hiroe Onaka, and Kosuke Yamazaki

Summary. A follow-up study to evaluate the course of treatment on the prognosis of individuals with an autistic disorder was conducted on subjects under treatment at the Child and Adolescent Psychiatry Clinic of Tokai University Hospital. Seventy-five patients fulfilled the criteria of having received more than 3 years of continuous outpatient treatment and being over 15 years of age as of April 1989. The results indicated that although the autistic child's innate disabilities including intelligence and capacity for communicative speech often remained in the moderate to severe categories of delay, the actual level of adjustment attained by the children had improved compared to the projections made based on the disabilities and in comparison to reports on "first generation" autistic children, with a large proportion of subjects showing fair levels of adjustment. This result is believed to reflect the positive effects of long-term continual and consistent treatment and the proper consideration provided by those involved with the subjects and the parents in particular. As a next step, the importance of appropriate medical institutions that function to maintain close cooperation with home, school, and workplace (workshop) was emphasized for bringing about further improvement in the prognosis for persons with an autistic disorder.

Key words. Autistic disorder—Behavior modification program—Drug therapy—Outcome—Longitudinal study

There have been substantial changes in the treatment of autistic disorder during the last half century since the first report by Kanner; they were brought about through changes in the concept of autistic disorder. Until the beginning of the 1970s, autistic disorder was considered to be an early from of schizophrenia or an emotional disorder caused by failure in the parent—child relationship. Treatment during this time included institutionalization and observing the course of illness or conducting acceptive play therapy without any schooling for such children. We have come to call the children of this treatment era "first generation" autistic children. Since the mid-1970s, autistic disorder has come to be recognized as a syndrome with multiple factors and is considered a type of developmental disorder. As in the case of mental retardation, early diagnosis, early treatment, and education are stressed.

Department of Psychiatry and Behavioral Science, Tokai University School of Medicine, Bohseidai, Isehara, Kanagawa 259-11, Japan

In Japan a compulsory education law for disabled children was enacted in 1979. Since then, schools for handicapped children have been founded nationwide. Given the substantial changes brought about through this development, we call children raised in this treatment environment "second generation" autistic children.

Most longitudinal follow-up studies on autistic children have focused on first generation autistic children. The social outcome has been poor, and results have not been encouraging, indicating no positive correlation between treatment and prognosis [1–6]. There have been few studies on second-generation autistic children, and it is of interest to determine if the prognosis is still as pessimistic under the present treatment environment. In particular, there have been almost no studies on the long-

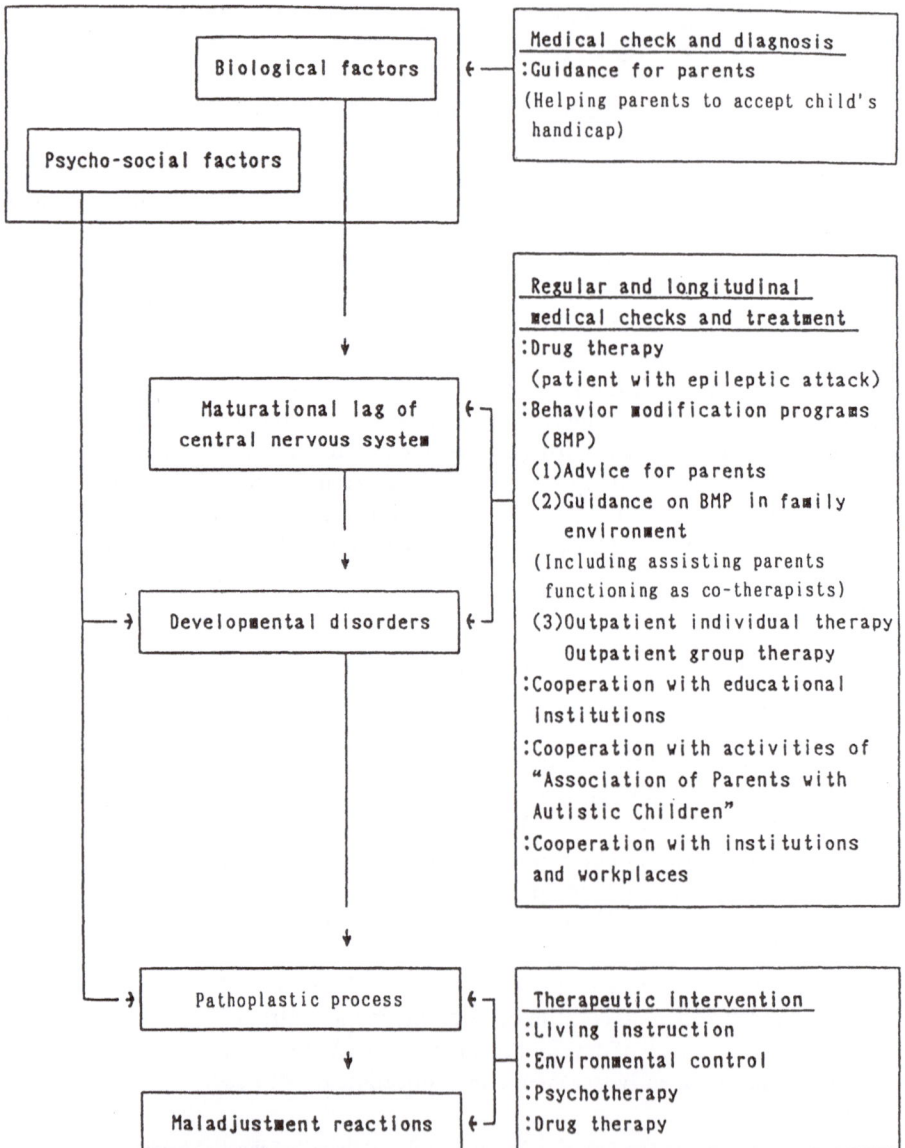

Fig. 1. Guidelines for Tokai University Hospital treatment and behavior modification programs (BMPs) for autistic children.

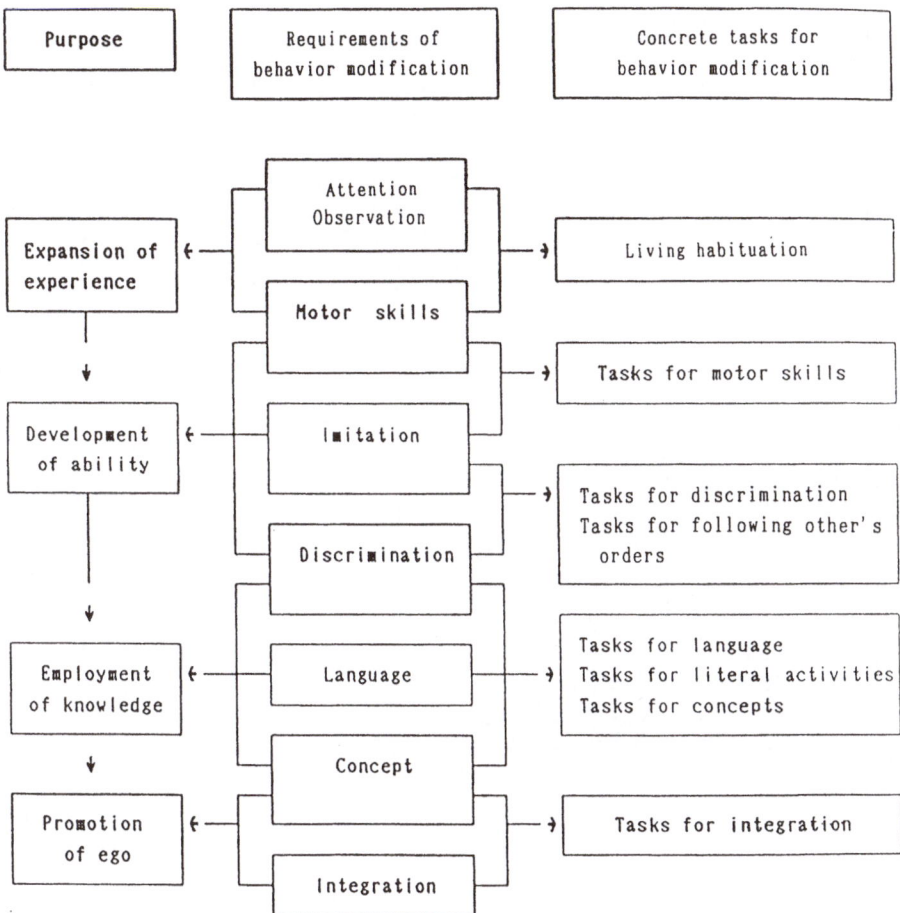

Fig. 2. Tokai University Hospital treatment and behavior modification programs for autistic children.

term prognosis of patients treated by a consistent, long-term therapy program conducted by a medical institution.

After establishment of the Child and Adolescent Psychiatric Clinic at Tokai University Hospital in 1975, we have provided autistic children and their families medical examinations and diagnosis, parental guidance, scheduled checkups and observation, and therapeutic intervention as required (e.g., drug therapy, psychotherapy, environmental control, living guidance). We have also been conducting treatment and behavior modification programs for autistic children, including advising parents, educating parents to function as co-therapists, guiding home study, and giving outpatient individual and group therapy. A further aspect of our function is cooperation with schools, places of employment, workshops, other institutions, and parent groups.

Figure 1 summarizes the guidelines for the treatment and behavior modification programs for autistic children of Tokai University Hospital. We have been treating autistic children according to these guidelines since 1975. The programs on which we place the most emphasis are outpatient individual therapy and outpatient group therapy. Through these programs, the parents become co-therapists and learn how to conduct behavior modification programs in the home.

Figure 2 and Table 1 outline the basic concept and actual contents of our behavior modification program, described elsewhere in detail [7]. The basic purpose of this

Table 1. Tokai University Hospital treatment and behavior modification programs for autistic children.

Concrete tasks for behavior modification	Family environment	Outpatient individual therapy	Outpatient group therapy
Living habituation	Eating meals Toilet training Dressing	Evaluation of level of learning tasks at home Formation of readiness to receive stimuli Coordination of eye and motor skills Montessori cylinder Puzzle box Picture puzzles	
Tasks for motor skills	Picture puzzles Lego blocks Behavioral imitation	Formation of responses toward verbal orders Lego blocks Matching Selection of picture cards	
Tasks for discrimination	Selection of real objects Selection of picture cards	Introduction to play Jigsaw puzzles Paper craft Paper mosaic drawing	
Tasks for following other's orders	Following verbal orders		Introduction to group Formation of group activities
Tasks for language	Learning of verbs	Comprehension of one's turn Person puzzles Seeking puzzles Fishing game	Comprehension of one's turn Person puzzles Seeking puzzles Phythmic athletic activity
Tasks for literal activities	Literal activities		
Tasks for concepts	Concept Comparison Position Number	Comprehension of rules Card play Sugoroku game Bingo game	Comprehension of rules Card play UNO game Bingo game
Tasks for integration	Self-expression Verbal Behavioral Living ability Home situation Social situation		Changing of roles Railway backgammon Shopping game Purchase game

program is the expansion of experience, development of ability, employment of knowledge, and promotion of ego. The goals of this program are achieved through concrete tasks.

The purpose of our present study was to evaluate the effect of the course of treatment on the prognosis of children with autistic disorder when employing a consistent, long-term therapy program conducted by a medical institution. It is also a follow-up study on second-generation autistic children.

Subjects and Methods

The subjects of the follow-up study were autistic children receiving care at the outpatient clinic of the Department of Psychiatry at Tokai University Hospital. The subjects selected for the study were those over 15 years old as of April 1989 who had been receiving more than 3 years of continuous treatment in our department. Over a 14-year period since its inception in 1975, we treated 661 children diagnosed as autistic. These were 270 children over 15 years old, but only 75 (69 boys, 6 girls) met our research criteria and were capable of being followed up. The average age at initial treatment was 9 years 7 months, and the average age at the time of this research was 18 years 10 months. The average length of outpatient treatment was 9 years 4 months.

The research method included an interview with the subject and family, and evaluation of the present levels of IQ, communicative speech, and adjustment as well as assessment of clinical symptoms, present situation, course of treatment, and parental cooperation. The data were obtained by the therapists in charge of the cases and were analyzed statistically by the chi-square (χ^2) test.

Results

Present Level of IQ

The subjects were classified into four levels of intelligence—normal to borderline IQ, mild retardation, moderate retardation, and severe retardation—using results (and estimations) primarily from the Suzuki-Binet IQ test as reference (Table 2). The results indicate that 13.3% have normal to borderline IQ, 14.7% mild retardation, 48.0% moderate retardation, and 24.0% severe retardation. The levels of IQ at the time these subjects began school were normal to borderline in 6.7%, mild retardation 6.7%, moderate retardation 41.3%, and severe retardation 45.3%. Comparing the figures, it

Table 2. IQ at the beginning of school and currently.

IQ	Beginning of school*	Currently*
Normal to borderline	5 (6.7%)	10 (13.3%)
Mild retardation	5 (6.7%)	11 (14.7%)
Moderate retardation	31 (41.3%)	36 (48.0%)
Severe retardation	34 (45.3%)	18 (24.0%)
Total*	75 (100%)	75 (100%)

* $P < 0.05$ for IQ at the beginning of school versus that currently in all categories.

can be said that the IQ levels had risen considerably overall, even though 72% remain in the realm of moderate or severe retardation.

Present Level of Communicative Speech

Levels of communicative speech were evaluated in terms of the following four categories: normal (adequate for age or capable of conversing with practically no inconvenience, in addition to an absence of unnatural inflections), mildly delayed and deviant (capable of conversing, albeit unnaturally, in a monotonous and stereotyped manner), moderately delayed and deviant (voices utterances with meaning, employs one- to two-word sentences whom voicing demands or in responses, although echolalia can also be observed), and severely delayed and deviant (lack of utterances with meaning, or if speech is present it is echolalic) (Table 3). In terms of the present level of communicative speech, the results indicated 10.7% were in the normal range, 38.7% in the mildly delayed deviant range, 45.3% in the moderately delayed deviant range, and 5.3% in the severely delayed and deviant range. When the subjects were beginning school, the figures were 0% in the normal range, 14.7% in the mildly delayed deviant range, 40.0% in the moderately delayed deviant range, and 45.3% in the severely delayed deviant range. These figures represent a clear indication that the level of communicative speech had improved. However, 50.6% of the subjects are still in the moderately or severely delayed deviant categories, and they can speak only two- to three-word sentences at best.

Present Level of Adjustment

Levels of adjustment were evaluated in terms of the following three categories with reference to the evaluation standards of Eisenberg [2] and Rutter et al. [5]: good adjustment (capable of an independent or close to independent existence appropriate for their age and leading normal lives at home, in school, or on the job); fair adjustment (capable of a certain degree of autonomy in a carefully controlled environment but prone to difficulty in life at home, school, or the workplace; requiring appropriate support for overcoming such difficulties); and poor adjustment (difficulty leading an autonomous existence, characterized by marked difficulties in life at home, school, or the workplace, requiring constant care or consistent support in a carefully controlled environment). As a result, 32% were found to show good adjustment, 44% fair adjustment, and 24% poor adjustment, indicating a definitely larger proportion of those with fair adjustment than with poor adjustment.

Table 3. Level of communicative speech at beginning of school and currently.

Speech	Beginning of school*	Currently*
Normal	0(0%)	8 (10.7%)
Mildly delayed	11 (14.7%)	29 (38.7%)
Moderately delayed	30 (40.0%)	34 (45.3%)
Severely delayed	34 (45.3%)	4 (5.3%)
Total	75 (100%)	75 (100%)

*$P < 0.001$ for all categories.

Table 4. Present IQ and adjustment.

IQ	Adjustment			
	Good	Fair	Poor	Total
Normal to borderline	10 (13.2%)	0 (0.0%)	0 (0.0%)	10 (13.3%)
Mild retardation	9 (12.0%)	0 (0.0%)	2 (2.7%)	11 (14.7%)
Moderate retardation	5 (6.7%)	24 (32.0%)	7 (9.3%)	36 (48.0%)
Severe retardation	0 (0.0%)	9 (12.0%)	9 (12.0%)	18 (24.0%)
Total	24 (32.0%)	33 (44.0%)*	18 (24.0%)*	75 (100.0%)

*$P < 0.05$ for the total fair adjustment group versus the total poor adjustment group.

Relation Between IQ and Adjustment

Analysis of the relation between levels of adjustment and IQ indicates that most of those exhibiting good adjustment had normal to borderline or mild retardation in terms of IQ (Table 4). On the other hand, the IQs of a large proportion of those showing poor adjustment were in the moderately or severely retarded range, and many of the subjects with fair adjustment fell into the moderately retarded category. It was notable that, although limited in number, there were some who had good adjustment despite their moderate retardation and some who had fair adjustment despite their severe retardation.

Relation Between the Level of Communicative Speech and Adjustment

Looking at the present adjustment in terms of level of communicative speech, it was seen that the level of communicative speech of all subjects exhibiting good adjustment were in the normal or mildly delayed and deviant range (Table 5). In contrast, most of those who exhibited poor adjustment fell into the moderately or severely delayed, deviant range. The levels of communicative speech among those showing fair adjustment varied.

Present Clinical Symptoms

When viewing the present clinical symptoms according to the level of adjustment, a lack of spontaneity or rapport, a bizarre or hypersensitive response, and preoccupation were seen in the subjects at all levels of adjustment, although the symptoms were most pronounced among those evaluated as having attained fair or poor levels of adjustment. Symptoms such as excitability, impulsiveness, hyperactivity, and epileptic seizures were rare among those exhibiting good adjustment but were frequently

Table 5. Levels of present communicative speech and adjustment.

Speech	Adjustment			
	Good	Fair	Poor	Total
Normal	8 (10.7%)	0 (0.0%)	0 (0.0%)	8 (10.7%)
Mildly delayed	16 (21.3%)	10 (13.3%)	3 (4.0%)	29 (38.7%)
Moderately delayed	0 (0.0%)	20 (26.7%)	14 (18.7%)	34 (45.3%)
Severely delayed	0 (0.0%)	3 (4.0%)	1 (1.3%)	4 (5.3%)
Total	24 (32.0%)	33 (44.0%)*	18 (24.0%)*	75 (100.0%)

*$P < 0.05$ comparing the fair and poor adjustment categorices.

Table 6. Present clinical symptoms according to the level of adjustment.

Symptom	Good (n = 24)	Fair (n = 33)	Poor (n = 18)	Total (n = 75)
Lack of spontaneity	7 (9.3%)	33 (44.0%)	17 (22.7%)	57 (76.0%)
Lack of rapport	6 (8.0%)	33 (44.0%)	18 (24.0%)	57 (76.0%)
Bizarre or hypersensitive response	5 (6.7%)	23 (30.7%)	18 (24.0%)	46 (61.3%)
Preoccupation	8 (10.7%)	22 (29.3%)	16 (21.3%)	46 (61.3%)
Excitability	4 (5.3%)	9 (12.0%)	9 (12.0%)	22 (29.3%)
Impulsiveness	0	3 (4.0%)	8 (10.7%)	11 (14.7%)
Epileptic seizure	1 (1.3%)	6 (8.0%)	4 (5.3%)	11 (14.7%)
Aggression	0	1 (1.3%)	7 (9.3%)	8 (10.7%)
Obsession	3 (4.0%)	2 (2.7%)	2 (2.7%)	7 (9.3%)
Hyperactivity	0	0	6 (8.0%)	6 (8.0%)
Self-injury	0	2 (2.7%)	3 (4.0%)	5 (6.7%)
Hallucinatory/delusional-like state	1 (1.3%)	0	2 (2.7%)	3 (4.0%)
Anxiety/fear	0	1 (1.3%)	1 (1.3%)	2 (2.7%)
Hypoactivity	0	0	1 (1.3%)	1 (1.3%)

observed among those with fair and poor levels of adjustment. Additionally, hallucinatory delusion-like states, although rare, were observed primarily among those exhibiting poor adjustment (Table 6).

Present Situation

A survey of the patients' present situation in terms of levels of adjustment revealed that 48% of all subjects were presently enrolled in school. Those exhibiting good adjustment overall were found in various educational facilities including ordinary high schools, high schools for handicapped children, and occupational schools. However, most of those in the fair and poor adjustment categories were enrolled in high schools for handicapped children. Most of the subjects in sheltered workshops were in the fair adjustment category, and those who were employed or in occupational training centers were in the good adjustment category. Furthermore, most of those living in institutions for the mentally handicapped and those who were unemployed and living at home were in the poor adjustment category (Table 7).

Therapeutic Course of the Behavior Modification Program

Age of placement in the behavior modification program, duration of therapy, content of therapy, and parental cooperation were evaluated in terms of the present level of adjustment. The results show that in terms of the initiative age of therapy, more than half the subjects were started in the program before age 9. There were significantly more subjects in this group who had fair to good levels of adjustment compared to those who entered the program after 15 years of age (Table 8).

In terms of duration in the program, most were enrolled for more than 6 years. Looking at the relation between the length of training and the level of adjustment, significantly larger numbers of subjects who underwent more than 9 years of training were exhibiting fair and good adjustment levels compared to those with 6 years or less

Table 7. Present situation and social adjustment.

Situation	Adjustment			
	Good (*n* = 24)	Fair (*n* = 33)	Poor (*n* = 18)	Total (*n* = 75)
Student	9 (12.0%)	17 (22.7%)	10 (13.3%)	36 (48.0%)
Ordinary high school	3 (4.0%)	0	0	3 (4.0%)
School for handicapped children	3 (4.0%)	16 (21.3%)	10 (13.3%)	29 (2.7%)
Occupational school	3 (4.0%)	1 (1.3%)	0	4 (5.3%)
University	0	0	0	0
Sheltered workshop	2 (2.7%)	12 (16.0%)	1 (1.3%)	15 (20.0%)
Employed	10 (13.3%)	0	0	10 (13.3%)
Institution for the mentally retarded	0	1 (1.3%)	5 (6.7%)	6 (8.0%)
Home, not employed	0	1 (1.3%)	2 (2.7%)	3 (4.0%)
Training center	2 (2.7%)	0	0	2 (2.7%)
Family business	1 (1.3%)	0	0	1 (1.3%)
Long-stay hospital	0	0	0	0 (0.0%)
Others	0	2 (2.7%)	0	2 (2.7%)

Table 8. Age at entry to behavior modification program and present level of adjustment.

Adjustment	No. of children, by age (years) at entry			
	9	9–15	15+	Total
Good	12 (16.0%)	10 (13.3%)	2 (2.7%)	24 (32.0%)
Fair	20 (26.7%)	13 (17.3%)	0	33 (44.0%)
Poor	8 (10.7%)	6 (8.0%)	4 (5.3%)	18 (24.0%)
Total	40 (53.3%)	29 (38.7%)	6 (8.0%)	75 (100.0%)

$P < 0.05$ for children 9 years old versus those 15+ years old, and children 9–15 years old versus those 15+ years old.

Table 9. Duration of training and present level of adjustment.

Adjustment	No. of patients, according to length of BMP training (years)				
	3–6	6–9	9–12	12+	Total
Good	4 (5.3%)	6 (8.0%)	7 (9.3%)	7 (9.3%)	24 (32.0%)
Fair	1 (1.3%)	14 (18.7%)	8 (10.7%)	10 (13.3%)	33 (44.0%)
Poor	5 (6.7%)	9 (12.0%)	2 (2.7%)	2 (2.7%)	18 (24.0%)
Total	10 (13.3%)	29 (38.7%)	17 (22.7%)	19 (25.3%)	75 (100.0%)

$P < 0.05$ for children in BMP 3–6 years versus those in BMP 9–12 years, and those in BMP 3–6 years versus those in BMP 12+ years.

of training. The difference was particularly significant between those showing fair and poor adjustments (Table 9).

In terms of the types of therapy, few subjects received advice or at-home training guidance alone, with more than 70% of the subjects receiving both at-home training guidance and outpatient individual or group therapy. A significantly larger proportion of these subjects fell into the fair or good categories than into the poor adjustment category (Table 10).

Table 10. Components of the behavior modification program and present level of adjustment.

Adjustment	(A) Advice for parents	(B) In-home training guidance	(C) In-home training guidance + outpatient individual therapy	(D) In-home training guidance + outpatient group therapy
Good ($n = 24$)	5 (6.7%)	2 (2.7%)	8 (10.7%)	9 (12.0%)
Fair ($n = 33$)	4 (5.3%)	1 (1.3%)	12 (16.0%)	16 (21.3%)
Poor ($n = 18$)	6 (8.0%)	4 (5.3%)	6 (8.0%)	2 (2.7%)
Total ($n = 75$)	15 (20.0%)	7 (9.3%)	26 (34.7%)	27 (36.0%)

$P < 0.01$ for (A) versus (D) and for (B) versus (D).

Table 11. Parental cooperation in the behavior modification program and present level of adjustment.

	No. with parental cooperation			
Adjustment	Good (A)	Fair (B)	Poor (C)	Total (D)
Good	22 (29.3%)	2 (2.7%)	0	24 (32.0%)
Fair	29 (38.7%)	2 (2.7%)	2 (2.7%)	33 (44.0%)
Poor	5 (6.7%)	9 (12.0%)	4 (5.3%)	18 (24.0%)
Total	56 (74.7%)	13 (17.3%)	6 (8.0%)	75 (100.0%)

$P < 0.001$ for (A) versus (B) and for (A) versus (C).

Parental cooperation in therapy is an important factor in effective implementation of the behavior modification program. In our follow-up survey, parental cooperation was evaluated in terms of three categories: good (capable of fully understanding the advice and guidance given with regard to therapy and of carrying out training in the home consistently in a manner appropriate to the situation); fair (capable of understanding the advice and guidance given and of carrying out training in the home although lacking in consistency); and poor (incapable of more than superficial understanding of advice and guidance and does not follow through in the program with consistency). Our study indicates that significantly larger numbers of subjects with good or fair adjustment had been given parental assistance (Table 11).

Therapeutic Course of Drug Therapy

Forty-four percent of the subjects received some form of drug therapy, principally those with a fair or poor level of adjustment. The initial age, duration, and type of drug therapy were evaluated in terms of the subjects' present level of adjustment. Most of those patients had been placed on drug therapy after age 9. In terms of adjustment level, drug therapy was started at age 15 or older for the fair adjustment subjects and at lower ages (but after age 9) for those in the poor adjustment category (Table 12).

Most subjects received less than 6 years of drug therapy (Table 13). The drugs employed were principally antiepileptics, major tranquilizers, cerebral metabolic enhancers, and hypnotics. Subjects presently in the fair and poor categories had in many cases been placed on antiepileptics and major tranquilizers (Table 14).

Table 12. Age at start of drug therapy and present level of adjustment.

Adjustment	~9 years	9–15 years	15+ years	Total
	No. of patients, by age at start of drugs			
Good	1 (1.3%)	4 (5.3%)	0	5 (6.7%)
Fair	2 (2.7%)	3 (4.0%)	9 (12.0%)	14 (18.8%)
Poor	1 (1.3%)	7 (9.3%)	6 (8.0%)	14 (18.7%)
Total	4 (5.3%)	14 (18.7%)	15 (20.0%)	33 (44.0%)

$P < 0.05$ for the group 9–15 years of age versus those 15+ years of age.

Table 13. Drug therapy and present level of adjustment.

Adjustment	~3 years	3–6 years	6–9 years	9–12 years	12+ years	Total
	No. of patients, by duration of drug therapy					
Good	2 (2.7%)	1 (1.3%)	1 (1.3%)	0	1 (1.3%)	5 (6.7%)
Fair	5 (6.7%)	6 (8.0%)	2 (2.7%)	0	0	13 (17.3%)
Poor	4 (5.3%)	7 (9.3%)	4 (5.3%)	0	0	15 (20.0%)
Total	11 (14.7%)	14 (18.7%)	7 (9.3%)	0	1 (1.3%)	33 (44.0%)

Table 14. Medication and present level of adjustment.

Adjustment	Antiepileptics	Major tranquilizers	Cerebral metabolic enhancers	Hypnotics
	No. of patients, by medication			
Good ($n = 24$)	2 (2.7%)	3 (4.0%)	3 (4.0%)	0
Fair ($n = 33$)	7 (9.3%)	7 (9.3%)	3 (4.0%)	1 (1.3%)
Poor ($n = 18$)	3 (4.0%)	12 (16.0%)	5 (6.7%)	4 (5.3%)
Total ($n = 75$)	12 (16.0%)	22 (29.3%)	11 (14.7%)	5 (6.7%)

Discussion

Therapeutic Course and General Outcome

The most notable result from our follow-up study was that the levels of adjustment were better than had been projected from the levels of intelligence and communicative speech despite the fact that 72% of our subjects fell into the moderate and severe categories with regard to disorder of intelligence. It was particularly true for the significant increase in the proportion of those who attained a fair adjustment level, compared to the results of previous studies, which had indicated a poor adjustment for large numbers of children. Our results depict a tendency found in common with recent follow-up studies [4, 8]. The factors giving rise to this change in prognosis cannot be accounted for in general terms, but perhaps the following can be said in this regard. The subjects in follow-up studies conducted in recent years [9], including our current study, are not first-generation autistic children—who were diagnosed as having a psychosis or an emotional disorders and so did not obtain appropriate treatment or education. Our subjects belong to the second-generation group of autistic children—in whom the disorder is recognized as a developmental disorder at an age when early diagnosis, early treatment, and education have become the norm. Most autistic children growing up during this era, almost without exception, have participated in early treatment programs and have received a school education, factors that may be regarded as giving rise to the improved prognosis. In addition to school education, we have been conducting at-home training as part of a consistent training program both during the school years and after graduation, with the parents functioning as co-therapists. Employing drug therapy as needed, we have been working together with family, school, and places of employment (workshops). We believe the results from this study indicate that the daily implementation of the behavior modification program for autistic children from early infancy to adulthood in the home improved the level of adjustment and was effective in maintaining that level. However, the subjects in the recent follow-up studies including ours are principally autistic adolescents, and the period for which they have been followed is short compared to the 30-year follow-up study of the first 11 cases of autism conducted by Kanner [3]. Therefore it is open to debate whether the findings obtained in this study will hold for the subjects into adulthood.

Symptomatological Outcome

With the approach of adolescence, autistic children may experience a worsening of clinical symptoms or come to manifest symptoms that were not seen previously, capable of affecting their levels of adjustment. Symptoms noted most frequently during adolescence compared to those seen during infancy or early school age include epileptic seizures, aggressiveness, self-injurious behavior, and panic. Obsessive-compulsive symptoms and hallucinatory delusion-like states are also seen at times. These findings were demonstrated in our follow-up study. We counter the symptoms that become more pronounced during adolescence by therapeutic intervention including drug therapy as required, and in most cases we have been successful in maintaining the level of adjustment the subjects had attained. With regard to hallucinatory delusion-like states, Petty et al. [10] noted a subgroup within the general autism category who develop schizophrenia, but our subjects presented a condition separate from schizophrenia. With regard to this issue, Rumsey et al. [11] reported negatively on the possibility of autism developing into schizophrenia through an evaluation of clinical outcomes in adults, but the question remains and requires further evaluation.

Factors Controlling Outcome

Intelligence, the capacity for communicative speech, the severity of the disorder, and school education have been cited as important factors controlling the outcome of autistic disorder. Our study has indicated a close relation between intelligence, the capacity for communicative speech, and level of adjustment. The importance of continuous, consistent, comprehensive medical care was also demonstrated to be an important factor that controls outcome. Traditionally in Japan there has been a strong tendency for autistic children to discontinue treatment at medical and guidance institutions once the child enters a school, shifting the site of training from the original facility to the school, to which the parents relegate the responsibility of training and education. Such subjects then were often returned to the medical institution or guidance institution when their problem behavior (e.g. panic, self-injury, aggressive behavior, or episodes of epileptic seizures) became pronounced as they grow older. Even though the subjects do return to the auspices of medical care, lack of a consistent treatment approach, considered the most important factor in the treatment of autistic children, has been the norm in Japan [12]. It is believed that for further improvement to be made on the prognosis of autistic disorder, close cooperation between appropriate medical institutions and the home, school, and workplace (workshop) is imperative, and medical institutions must fulfill their function from the standpoint of comprehensive medical care.

Conclusion

Although the autistic child's innate disabilities show some alleviation over the course of development, the children often remain moderately to severely retarded. The subjects in our follow-up study had achieved levels of adjustment far beyond projections based on their levels of communicative speech and intelligence in light of reports made on first-generation autistic children. Most of our subjects demonstrated a fair level of adjustment. This result is believed to be a reflection of our consistent long-term treatment approach with emphasis on day-to-day training in the home, parallel training and education in school, and comprehensive care in medical institutions.

References

1. DeMyer MK, Barton S, DeMyer WF, et al (1973) Prognosis in autism—a follow-up study. J Autism Child Schizophr 3:199–246
2. Eisenberg L (1956) The autistic child in adolescence. Am J Psychiatry 112:607–612
3. Kanner L (1971) Follow-up study of eleven autistic children; originally reported in 1943. J Autism Child Schizophr 1:119–145
4. Lotter V (1974) Social adjustment and placement of autistic children in Middlesex: a follow-up study. J Autism Child Schizophr 4:11–32
5. Rutter M, Greenfield D, Lockyer L (1967) A five to fifteen year follow-up study of infantile psychosis. II. Social and behavioural outcome. Br J Psychiatry 113:1183–1199
6. Wakabayashi S, Mizuno M (1975) A study on the prognosis in the autistic children. Jpn J Child Psychiatry 16:177–196
7. Hayashi M, Takamura I, Yamazaki K (1992) Autism—its medical treatment and social support. Jpn J Clin Psychiatry 21:9–18
8. Gillberg C, Steffenburg S (1987) Outcome and prognostic factors in infantile autism and similar conditions: a population-based study of 46 cases followed through puberty. J Autism Dev Disord 17:273–287
9. Kobayashi R (1985) A clinical study on the mental development and the clinical course of autistic children. Psychiatr Neurol Jpn 87:546–582
10. Petty LK, Ornitz EM, Michelman JD, et al (1984) Autistic children who become schizophrenic. Arch Gen Psychiatry 41:129–135
11. Rumsey JM, Rapaport JL, Sceery WR (1985) Autistic children as adults: psychiatric, social and behavioral outcomes. J Am Acad Child Psychiatry 24:465–473
12. Oshima M (1984) Medical and educational care after admission to elementary school for the autistic children. Psychiatr Neurol Jpn 86:53–66

Review of Learning Disability Studies in Japan

Masanori Hanada

Summary. Special educational studies have been conducted on children with learning disabilities since the 1960s in the United States. These children have poor school records even though they are intellectually normal without mental retardation and have no visual, hearing, or motor impairment. They have no special problems at home and have had a normal growth history. In Japan, the definition and concept of learning disability have not been established, although the educational field began to pay attention to learning disabilities some years ago. The history, opinions of experts, and studies of learning disability are described here regarding both medical and educational aspects.

Key words. Learning disability—Reading-writing disability—Hyperkinetic—Attention deficit disorder—Minimal brain damage

Introduction

Special educational studies have been conducted in the United States since the 1960s on children with learning disabilities (LD) who had poor school records though intellectually normal. They are not mentally retarded and have no visual, hearing, or motor impairment. Moreover, there are no special problems in the home environment, and the growth history is normal.

In Japan, the number of children regarded as having a reading/writing disability (RWD) has been small because of the characteristics of the Japanese language, that is, the combination of kana (Syllabary characters) and kanji (ideograms). In addition, RWD is' sometimes considered an educational problem rather than a medical problem.

The educational field began to pay attention to LD some years ago. In 1992 the Japanese Ministry of Education designated nine primary schools to cooperate in research of instruction methods for students with LD or with difficulty in learning that resembles an LD. The term LD has come to be been used in various places and is now widely known.

Department of Neuropsychiatry, Kinki University School of Medicine, 377-2 Ohno-Higashi, Osaka-Sayama, Osaka 589, Japan

The definition and concept of LD have not been established, however. We describe the history of LD, introduce opinions and studies from the medical and educational aspects, and present our personal views on LD.

History

Before the concept of LD emerged there was recognition of hyperkinetic children, attention deficit disorder, and minimal brain damage (MBD). LD seemed to be the umbrella under which these problems could reside. In terms of learning ability in these individuals, reading and writing abilities are decreased and therefore, RWD should also be reviewed here.

Reading/Writing Disability

Historically, RWD is the oldest recognized disability in our modern world. Kussmaul [1] reported cases of RWD in 1877 and called the symptoms observed (due to impaired cerebral function in adults) "word blindness" (*Wordblindheit*). In 1896 Morgan [2] reported a 14-year-old boy who could read each letter but not words and had impaired dictation as well. Morgan called this condition "congenital word blindness."

In Japan Kobi [3] was the first to report a case of congenital word blindness in 1957. Since then, various cases have been reported and diagnosed as specific dyslexia, specific reading disability, congenital symbol amblyopia, or strephosymbolia. Thus the definition and concept became varied. However, because writing and speech are learned and mastered after birth, it may be appropriate to call this condition developmental alexia and agraphia.

When RWD is interpreted in a broad sense, the following groups emerge:

1. Those in whom RWD is considered to be congenital because of the absence of findings suggesting definite cerebral damage
2. Those in whom the personal history suggests cerebral damage
3. Those with neurological findings suggesting definite cerebral damage
4. Those with mental retardation
5. Those who exhibit behavioral problems such as restlessness and difficulty with concentration of attention
6. Those in whom RWD seems to be secondary to environmental problems

Reading/writing disability, in a narrow sense, may be characterized by impaired cerebral function and impaired symbolic function as is observed with adult alexia. Wernicke [4] classified adult alexia as (1) cortical, (2) subcortical, and (3) transcortical. Adult alexia can be also classified as literal alexia and verbal alexia or, according to the site of damage, as occipital alexia and parietal alexia. Occipital alexia is visual agnostic alexia (pure alexia) and primarily literal; it is characterized by poor copying and the absence of impaired dictation or spontaneous writing. With parietal alexia, copying is good without visual agnosia, but dictation and spontaneous writing are poor.

Johnson and Myklebust [5] classified dyslexia as visual and auditory types. They explained that the former is characterized by reversals or errors in order and the latter by discrimination of read sounds.

Concerning the pathogenesis, some researchers suggest that a brain lesion causes adult alexia, whereas others believe that an organic (but not regional) cause is present. There are two major explanations for RWD: impairment of all mental functions or impairment of instrumental functions. There is also a case report suggesting the importance of hereditary disposition and an association with autosomal dominant inheritance. In 1962 Kuromaru et al. [6] reported a family line with hereditary developmental alexia and agraphia. In recent years, alexia has been increasingly considered to be a symptom of LD due to perinatal abnormality.

Orton [7] reported that unbalanced lateralization of handedness, dominant eye or foot, and ambidexterity or left-handedness are frequently observed in those with RWD. He attributed these findings to abnormal cerebral dominance and suggested that inadequate cerebral laterality causes abnormal handedness or impaired writing and speech. Goody and Reinhold [8] reported that cerebral function is originally asymmetrical and differs between the dominant and recessive hemispheres; abnormality in lateralization in the dominant hand, eye, or foot or RWD develops when cerebral function does not differentiate asymmetrically. Thus there is a close association among abnormality in handedness, dominant eye or foot, reading and writing ability, and inadequate differentiation of asymmetrical cerebral function.

Abnormal perception of the order of letters, such as strephosymbolia, seems to be associated with impairment of the visual space. It suggests the association between RWD and Gerstmann's syndrome. Kuromaru et al. [6] and Anzial et al. [9] discussed the association with Gerstmann's syndrome. Detailed evaluation of right and left disorientation and spatial constructional impairment is necessary, as they are regarded as parietal lobe symptoms of the dominant hemisphere.

There are many reported cases of RWD in Western countries but relatively few in Japan. Makita [10] reported that the incidence of dyslexia in Japan is less than 10% that in Western countries, and the literature on it is scanty. He detected dyslexia in 89 (0.97%) of 9195 children based on a questionnaire table checked by teachers. In addition, according to the character type, dyslexia of kana decreased from the third grade of primary school, reaching zero at the fourth grade. In contrast, dyslexia of kanji increased from about the third grade of primary school. As mentioned above, the low incidence of dyslexia in Japan may be associated with the specificity of the language (i.e., the combination of kana, or syllabary characters, and kanji, or ideograms). Reading the combinations of 48 kana symbols and 1850 kanji characters is more difficult than reading the combinations of 26 roman letters. However, visual perception of kanji is easy, and there are no kana symbols that have mirror images with completely different sounds (e.g., p ↔ q, b ↔ d). Unlike roman letters that are pronounced in different ways (e.g., a → [a], [e], [ei]), there is only one pronunciation for each kana symbol. With kana, oral language corresponds to written language. When discrimination and perception of sounds are correct, conversion to letters is easy. The variety of sounds that should be discriminated is small compared with that in Western languages.

Hyperkinetic Children

Hyperkinesis in children has attracted attention since about 1902 as a behavioral characteristic of cerebral damage, acute disorders, and various conditions suspected to be associated with cerebral damage. In 1918 there was an epidemic of encephalitis, and affected children showed restless behavior. In affected children without definite cerebral damage, evaluation of their problems prenatally suggested slight cerebral damage. After this epidemic, the opinion that the restless behavioral pattern is associated with cerebral damage became widely accepted.

With this background, Pasamanick and Knobloch [11] in 1959 introduced the term "minimal cerebral damage" (MCD) to pediatric neurology. They noted that careful examination sometimes reveals delay or distortion in the process of behavioral development even in children without marked behavioral abnormalities or neurological signs in who cerebral damage during pregnancy or the perinatal period is suspected. These children sometimes showed slight neurological signs that could not be detected by routine neurological examination. Based on this clinical exprience, they speculated that MCD is present and causes slight delay or distortion in behavioral development. Since 1960 MCD has been used for children with normal intelligence who show abnormal behavior or a specific learning disability. However, at symposiums held in England and the United States in 1962 and 1963, the term "minimal cerebral damage" was considered to be inappropriate, and the use of "minimal cerebral dysfunction" (MCD) was recommended.

In 1986, Eisenberg [12] used "hyperkinetic syndrome" to describe children for whom MCD had conventionally been used. They did not associate restless behavior with cerebral damage alone but, rather, considered it to be a result of overlapping of various problems including cerebral damage. Suzuki [13]. cautioned against using MCD as a "dumping place" diagnosis and classified the condition into the following six categories:

1. Minor motor disorders
2. Hyperkinetic behavior
3. Communication disorders
4. Perceptual disorders
5. Mental deficiency
6. Convulsive disorders

Concerning "soft neurological signs," which are conjunctive diagnostic signs in such children, Garfield [14] performed the following eight motion maintenance tests, considering that children with cerebral damage cannot maintain a certain movement or posture: (1) maintaining eye closure; (2) tongue protrusion with the eyes closed: (3) tongue protrusion with the mouth open; (4) gaze of the lateral visual field; (5) maintaining an open mouth; (6) gazing at the examiner's nose during perimeter movement; (7) backward bending of the head at the time of sensory examination; and (8) pronunciation of "Ah—." In 1970 Touwen and Prechtl [15] examined the subjects in the standing position and for gait, thereby establishing a method to objectively evaluate soft neurological signs in terms of movement.

In Japan Kuromaru et al. [16] in 1964 performed (1) a rotation test; (2) an eyeball test; (3) a two-point simultaneous stimulation test; and (4) a slight involuntary movement test in children aged 3-8 years who had been born at term with a normal delivery. They compared the results with those from age-matched immature children and children with mental retardation, head injury, epilepsy, or schizophrenia. In 1967 Kuromaru et al. [17] investigated signs in neonates, 3-year-old children, and school children in whom these was slight cerebral damage during the neonatal period. These authors suggested that behavioral characteristics cannot be evaluated simply as intellectual impairment or at the purely psychological level, but that they are associated with impaired movement and behavior such as restlessness or distractibility. In addition, they speculated that mental retardation is typically caused by damage in the cerebral cortex, but the cerebral damage in these children is present in the old cortex centered in the basal ganglia.

Minimal cerebral dysfunction in children was first discussed in Japan during a panel discussion at the 71st meeting of the Japanese Pediatric Society held in 1968. The content of the discussion was later published in the *Journal of Pediatric Practice* (Volume 31). That same year, Suzuki [13] described the concept, diagnosis, and prognosis of MCD. Ohtahara [18] performed an electroencephalographic (EEG) study of MCD syndrome and reported (1) diffuse slow-wave dysrhythmia; (2) juvenile occipital slow waves; (3) abnormal basal waves, such as hypersynchronous α; (4) 14- and 6-cps positive spikes; (5) 6-cps phantom waves; and (6) anterior θ waves, suggesting the importance of waveforms to indicate diencephalon dysfunction. In 1969 Nagahata [19] reported MCD syndrome in children, and Fukuyama [20] reported the basic concept of MCD syndrome. In 1976 a special issue (Soft Neurological Signs and Minor Anomalies) was published in *Pediatric Medicine* (Vol. 9). In that issue, Okada and Hanada [21] reported that development should be considered constantly when the neurological examination is performed in children; they also noted the importance of the fact that soft neurological signs differ according to the child's development. At the 18th meeting of the Japanese Society of Pediatric Neurology (1976), a symposium on soft neurological signs, with their evaluation and importance to pediatric neurology, was held.

Learning Disabilities

The educational field has long been aware of children with normal intellectual ability, visual acuity, and hearing for whom good school records are expected but for whom the results of learning are poor. This condition began to attract attention as learning disability (LD) in 1960. Myklebust [22] established the concept of LD. He speculated that impaired learning ability is caused by central neurological factors, although behavioral problems, not neurological signs, are evident. He defined LD as follows:

1. Impaired learning ability
2. Absence of mental retardation
3. Absence of impaired sensory organs
4. Absence of marked motor disturbance

In 1968 the *Journal of Learning Disabilities* was started in the United States. In Japan Yamaguchi [23] referred to LD in "Three cases of clumsy children" in 1973. He reported that there are children with neurological problems among those who were diagnosed as having emotional disturbance due to isolation, restlessness, peculiar habits, or difficulty with group activities, indicating misdiagnosis. In 1975 Suzuki [24] reported that LD is essentially a neurological disorder and a manifestation of "minimal cerebral damage," but damage in the child's cerebrum that shows incomplete functional differentiation does not cause permanent or irreversible impairment, as observed in the adult brain, and is adequately compensated by cerebral elasticity. In 1982 Ohkudo et al. [25] reported that brain waves in children with LD show a high incidence of juvenial occipital slow waves, 6- and 14-Hz positive spikes, prolonged spindles, seizure waves, and slowing. In 1982 Uemura [26] introduced a practical screening test for LD in children. In 1981 Tatsunuma et al. [27] carried out an epidemiological survey of children with reading difficulty in Miyakojima and demonstrated the low incidence of this problem in Japan, as had been expected. Saito et al. [28] reported in detail two children with a delay in constructional ability and slowness in motion despite normal linguistic ability.

There have been only a few studies in the field of childhood and adolescence psychiatric medicine that used the term LD in Japan. It is partly because LD children rarely are seen by the psychiatric department since psychiatric symptoms are not marked.

Psychiatric Diagnostic Criteria of LD

The disorder called hyperkinetic reaction of childhood in DSM-II was redefined in DSM-III as an attention deficit disorder. The disorder was subclassified as an attention deficit disorder with hyperactivity (ADDH) or without hyperactivity (ADD). The former corresponds to the hyperkinetic reaction of childhood classification in DSM-II. In addition, DSM-III-R in 1987 included this disorder as an academic skills disorder under the category of specific developmental disorders and subclassified it as developmental arithmetic disorder, developmental expressive writing disorder, and developmental reading disorder.

In contrast, the World Health Organization (WHO) International Classification of Disease 9 (ICD-9) in 1979 classified this condition as hyperkinetic syndrome of childhood and specific delay in development. The latter includes developmental dyslexia, dyscalculia, developmental speech or language disorder, clumsiness syndrome, and dyspraxia syndrome. ICD-10 in 1990 proposed the definition of specific developmental disorders of speech and language. These disorders included specific speech articulation disorder, expressive language disorder, and receptive language disorder, whereas specific developmental disorders of scholastic skills included specific reading disorder, specific spelling disorder, and specific disorder of arithmetic skills.

Each of these classification methods has advantages and disadvantages. ICD-10 provides the most detailed diagnostic guidelines and shows the following five findings as basic requirements for the diagnosis of specific developmental impairment:

1. Specific academic ability is impaired to a clinically significant degree.
   a. The severe form of the disorder is expected to be observed in 3% of school children.
   b. Developmental delay or deviation in speech of language is observed before school attendance.
   c. Associated disorders such as disturbance in attention, emotion, or behavior are observed.
   d. A qualitative abnormality that is not observed during normal development is present.
   e. The problem cannot be immediately alleviated even by changes in the educational method or educational environment.
2. The disorder is specific and cannot be explained by mental retardation.
3. The disorder is developmental and observed during an early stage of education.
4. There are no external factors that are adequate causes of difficulty in learning.
5. The disorder is not directly due to an uncorrected visual or hearing impairment.

Recent Problems of LD

The Ministry of Education carried out a survey of LD via boards of education. They reported in July 1991 that there are school children with learning difficulty; but the definition, diagnostic criteria, evaluation criteria, and diagnostic methods have not been standardized, and active basic studies are necessary. In March 1992 they reported again that the central definition of LD is accepted by most people, but its details are still questioned. Moreover, some of the methods used to correct an LD can be performed in the ordinary classroom or in a special class, but others require individual instruction or group instruction (with just a few students).

An association of LD children and their parents was established on February 11, 1990, and the group presented a written request consisting of the following six items to the Ministry of Welfare on August 29, 1991:

1. Establishment of an acceptable definition of LD
2. Enforcement of a survey of the present status of LD in Japan
3. Establishment of a system for early detection
4. Establishment of a system for early treatment and education
5. Establishment of a system for lifetime treatment, education, and consultation
6. Enlightenment activities

In 1985 the Japanese Society of Child and Adolescent Psychiatry examined LD in a special issue of the *Japanese Journal of Child and Adolescent Psychiatry*, which contained the papers shown in Table 1. In addition, a panel discussion on LD was held at the 26th meeting of the Japanese Society of Child and Adolescent Psychiatry (Table 2). In those days, however, little attention was paid to LD by the medical field. In more recent years, since LD has increasingly attracted attention, a special issue on LD appeared again in the *Japanese Journal of Child and Adolescent Psychiatry* (Table 3). This journal contained the concept of LD, the nosological position, and the neuropsychological approach as general remarks; an original article; and discussions

Table 1. Special issue: learning disabilities: *Japanese Journal of Child and Adolescent Psychiatry* 26(4), 1985.

Makita K: The attitudes of child psychiatrists dealing with learning disabilities and allied conditions
Hanada M, Ueda T: On the concept of learning disabilities
Yamaguchi T: Apropos of learning disabilities
Morinaga R: A psychological approach to learning disabilities
Nakane H: Learning disability and hyperkinetic syndrome—based on a questionnaire concerning the diagnosis and treatment of hyperkinetic syndrome

---

Table 2. Special issue: learning disabilities: 26th Congress of The Society of Child and Adolescent Psychiatry at Kanagawa Kenritsu Ongakudou, October 1985.

Nakane A: Learning disabilities and emotional disturbance
Yamaguchi T: Apropos of learning disabilities
Shirataki S: A developmental neurological approach to learning disabilities
Morinaga R: A psychological approach to learning disabilities

Table 3. Special issue: learning disorders: *Japanese Journal of Child and Adolescent Psychiatry* 34(4), 1993.

General remarks
    Yamazaki K: Transition in the concept of learning disorders
    Kurita H: Nosological position of learning disorders in developmental disorders
    Shirataki S: A neuropsychological approach to learning disabilities
Original article
    Nakane A: A clinical approach to learning disabilities as memory disability
Discussions
    Kamiide H
    Nagahata M
    Morinaga R

by Kamiide on the aspects of the welfare of the LD child, by Nagahata reporting as a doctor at a children's hospital, and by Morinaga who observes LD students at a college. Each presentation was primarily a personal view.

For the present, the concept of LD should be established; and studies on statistics, detection methods, and approaches to treatment should be performed. Subsequently, the concept of LD should be evaluated and revised if necessary and additional studies carried out to obtain a consensus among staff in the medical and educational fields and at child welfare facilities.

References

1. Kussmaul A (1877) Disturbance of speech. Cyclopedia Pract Med 14:581–591
2. Morgan WP (1896) A case of congenital word blindness. BMJ 2:1378–1389
3. Kobi I (1957) A case of congenital word blindness. 58:825–859
4. Wernicke C (1885) Die neueren Arbeiten über Aphasie. Fortschr Med 3:824–830
5. Johnson DJ, Myklebust HR (1964) Learning disabilities. Grune and Stratton, Orlando
6. Kuromaru S, Okada S, Hanada M (1962) Developmental alexia and agraphia. Pediatr Med 25:853–858
7. Orton ST (1925) Word-blindness in school children. Arch Neurol Psychiatry 14:581–615
8. Goody W, Reinhold M (1961) Congenital dyslexia and asymmetry of cerbral function. Brain 84:231–241
9. Anzai S, Iwata A, Ikeda A (1966) Reading-writing disability in a 6 year-old case. Psychiatr Neurol Jpn 68:627–641
10. Makita K (1968) The rarity of reading disability in Japanese children. J Orthopsychiatry 38:599–614
11. Pasamanick B, Knobloch H (1959) Syndrome of minimal cerebral damage in infancy. JAMA 170:1338–1387
12. Eisenberg L (1966) The management of the hyperkinetic child. Dev Med Child Neurol 8:593–599
13. Suzuki M (1968) Minimal cerebral damage. Prog Med 67:617–621
14. Garfield JC (1964) Motor impersistence in normal and brain-damaged children. Neurology 14:623–630
15. Touwen BCL, Prechtl HFR (1970) The neurological examination of the child with minor nervous dysfunction. Clin Dev Med 38:1–91
16. Kuromaru S, Okada S, Hanada M (1964) Soft neurological sign on children. Psychiatr Neurol Paediatr Jpn 4:69–77
17. Kuromaru S, Okada S, Hanada M (1967) The relationship between perinatal disturbances and abnormal behavior. Psychiatr Neurol Paediatr Jpn 7:212–219

18. Ohtahara T (1968) Electroencephalographic study on minimal cerebral damage. Pediatr Med 31:1233–1247
19. Nagahata M (1969) Minimal cerebral damage in children. Pediatr Rev 2:637–658
20. Fukuyama Y (1974) Basic concept of minimal brain damage. Pediatr Med 37:135–147
21. Okada S, Hanada M (1976) Soft neurological sign in cerebral function and its development. Pediatr Rev 9:161–180
22. Myklebust HR (1968) Learning disabilities. Grune and Stratton, Orlando, FL
23. Yamaguchi T (1973) Three cases of clumsy children. Jpn J Child Psychiatry 14:237–253
24. Suzuki M (1975) Diagnosis of learning disability. Pediatrics 16:607–619
25. Ohkudo O, Ogawa K, Hibio S (1982) Psychiatr Neurol Paediatr Jpn 22:27–32
26. Uemura K (1982) Diagnosis of learning disability. Brain Dev 14:294–298
27. Tatunuma T, Ichinowatari N, Ohki T (1981) Epidemiological research of dyslexia in Miyakozima. Boueidai Med J 6:275–278
28. Saito H, Imabashi S, Iida H (1982) Two cases of non-verbal learning disorder. Psychiatr Neurol Pediatr Jpn 22:127–134

Part 2

Infant Psychiatry

Infant Psychiatry: Review of Recent Trends

Sadaaki Shirataki

Summary. Infant psychiatry has developed rather recently as a subspecialty that is concerned with clinical problems in the mental development of infants. We have limited knowledge of the clinical problems and normal mental development during these years and must still depend on other academic fields such as developmental psychology, developmental neurology, pediatrics, and obstetrics. The aim of this chapter is to review recent trends in infant psychiatry by focusing on several relevant topics. In this review, the field of infant psychiatry is divided into two parts: theoretical and clinical (practical) aspects. In the theoretical aspect, recent progress in understanding the normal development of (1) cognitive (including the issue of "state"), (2) motor, and (3) emotional and social functions of newborn and young infants is described. The issue of continuity and discontinuity of development from infancy to later developmental periods is also described. In the clinical aspect, the following topics are discussed: (1) infant health checkups at 1.5 and 3.0 years; (2) prognosis for high-risk infants; (3) classification of infant psychiatric disorders; and (4) intervention and therapeutic methods for infant psychiatric disorders. Strong emphasis is placed on the need in both the theoretical and clinical areas of infant psychiatry to take a prospective rather than a retrospective stance. Such a stance enables us to consider the relation of infant development to later developmental periods in the life cycle.

Key words. Infant psychiatry—Recent trends—Theoretical aspect—Clinical aspect

Infant psychiatry has developed rather recently as a subspecialty and concerns clinical problems in the mental development of infants 0 to 3 years of age. American child psychiatrists (most of them are child psychoanalysts) have played a leading role in the establishment of a worldwide association (WAIPAD) for those concerned with infant and child mental health; the process by which the association was established has been reported in detail by Okonogi [1]. In Japan as well, much attention has been paid recently to the issue of the mental health of infants, irrespective of whether the term infant psychiatry is used. Even more attention should be paid by psychiatrists involved with infant psychiatry, as infant psychiatry can answer important questions in psychiatry in general, such as the causal mechanism of psychiatric disease, the

Department of Psychiatry and Neurology, Kobe University School of Medicine, 7-5-2 Kusunoki-Cho, Chuo-Ku, Kobe 650, Japan nature–nurture controversy regarding development, the continuity–discontinuity problem in development, and the predictability of future development according to the early condition of young infants. In this sense, Rutter [2] has advocated "developmental psychiatry."

What are the major elements of infant psychiatry? The answer may become clearer when we consider the characteristic features of infant existence. Infants have the following characteristics.

1. They are on the point of becoming a human being with a sociopsychological existence; in other words, they still have many of the characteristics of being a simple biological being.
2. They undergo a long period of complete dependence on the mother (or other caregiving person), which is unique to humans.

To understand these features in terms of infant psychiatry we must use knowledge gained in a mumber of scientific disciplines, including developmental psychology, developmental neurology, pediatrics, and obstetrics. In this sense, infant psychiatry constitutes a interdisciplinary field.

The purpose of this chapter is to review the recent trends in infant psychiatry, which of course is a monumental task. Therefore I limit the topics covered to several selected areas. The reader is referred to the introductory paper by Okonogi [1] for a more comprehensive discussion of infant psychiatry.

Theoretical Aspects of Infant Psychiatry

"State" of Newborn Infants

It has been acknowledged that newborn infants are equipped with a rather rich complement of cognitive and motor activity. They exhibit high-quality input functioning, information processing, and output functioning. Their functioning, however, has certain limits in terms of its availability, in contrast to adult functioning. That is, their input–output relation—information processing—can function only in a certain state, and they are greatly limited to this state.

The concept of "state" was first introduced by Wolff [3] and Prechtl [4], who subgrouped behaviors shown by the neonate; later, however, it was shown that the state of the infant can be used to subgroup the possible modes of brain functioning. Prechtl [4] subgrouped all states into five categories: State 1, eyes closed, regular respiration, no movements; State 2, eyes closed, irregular respiration, no gross movements; State 3, eyes open, no gross movements; State 4, eyes open, gross movements, no crying; State 5, eyes open or closed, crying. He showed that a different input-output relation can exist in each state.

The state alterations (state cycling) are controlled by the central nervous system (CNS), and state cycling can change according to the development of the CNS and may be disturbed if the CNS is affected. Wolff [3] recognized State 3 as "alert inactive," when newborns show their highest attentiveness toward the surrounding world. He has also found that the amount of time occupied by State 3 (alert inactivity) and State 4 (alert activity) within 24 hours can change at around 2 to 3 months of age. That is, the neural system devoted to cognitive activity drastically changes its mode of functioning at this point, which is said to be a point of discontinuity in neural development during early infancy.

The state concept so far outlined has contributed to an alteration in the past, fixed thinking that newborn and suckling infants should be viewed as reflex machines that respond only to incoming sensory stimuli. They are now seen as young infants in whom an important characteristic is spontaneous dynamics.

Cognitive and Motor Development

Cognitive Development

It has been recognized that newborns and young infants can differentiate incoming stimuli. One report [5] stated that newborns can discriminate the odor of their own mother from that of others, and other reports noted that different sensory modalities can be integrated by the newborn. Papousek [6] reported that classic conditioning is certainly possible in newborns, and Lipsitt [7] reported that habituation is possible.

Piaget had devised the terms "sensorimotor phase" and "preoperational phase" for the first few years after birth to describe cognitive development, and he postulated that infants of this age can recognize only their own subjective and personal world (egocentric world) instead of the real environment. Gibson [8] argued, however, that the environment the infant is recognizing is close to the real world, a concept called the "ecological theory of direct perception."

Motor Development

The process of walking is probably the most well studied among the many motor developmental stages. It is a sequential progression of motor milestones, such as neonatal head fixation, unaided sitting at around 6 months, rolling up and down, aided standing up, unaided walking, and so on. This sequential order of milestones is common to the wide variety of cultures in the world. On the other hand, the exact age at which each milestone is reached depends on the cultural environment. Because of the strictness of the sequential order, the latter can be applied to the clinical differentiation of abnormal motor development from normal development.

It is of theoretical interest to establish a sound developmental concept using motor development as an example. How does primitive walking during the neonatal period interrelate with unassisted walking, an ability attained at around 1 year of age? Is primitive walking during the neonatal period a precursor of the later appearing self-walking? Traditionally, the answer has been that many primitive reflexes during the neonatal period are suppressed by an inhibitory system, which becomes increasingly active with the development of the cortical substrates of the brain. Currently, we know that those primitive reflexes, after disapearance, can be elicited again under certain conditions during a later developmental period and even during adulthood.

Thelen et al. [9] has argued that neonatal primitive walking never disapears, but that it becomes difficult to elicit because of infants' remarkable increase in body weight and the progress in their ability to maintain a vertical position. These changes make it difficult for the infant's legs to support the total body. In this regard, I believe that Prechtl [10] is correct to say that true discontinuity in motor development exists between 2 and 3 months of postnatal life. It has long been maintained that CNS development exhibits its discontinuity at the time of birth. The advances in medical instrumentation, such as the ultrasound device used to monitor the fetus, has allowed us to observe fetal movements directly. As a result, we know about the motor skills repertoire of both the fetus and the newborn, and that the two are almost identical [11]. On the other hand, the CNS exhibits a remarkable qualitative difference at 2 to 3 months of age, when infants begin to develop an antigravity posture in their motor development.

The development of fetal motility has long been misunderstood because we could not observe it directly. Modern technological development has thus made it possible to recognize the actual motor development, not only during the newborn period but during the fetal months. Hence we now understand the complete process of motor development through the fetal, neonatal, and suckling periods.

Emotional and Social Development

Development of the Mother–Infant Relationship

The question of how newborns become attached to their care-giving, security-providing person has been answered in different ways in the past. The view that the infants become attached to their mother through repeated breastfeeding was the most dominant theory (secondary drive theory), but Bowlby [12] negated it. Although a student of Freud, he questioned the secondary drive theory because it did not explain the real situation in which the attachment of the infant was established with the mother. While in the process of questioning this theory, Bowlby was introduced to the work of ethologist K. Lorenz. Bowlby thus developed the "component instinctual responses theory," in which the concept of "attachment" is the crucial key issue. He believed that infants are born equipped with attachment behaviors as preparatory means for establishing attachment relationships.

Attachment behaviors by infants and the responsiveness by the mother make possible the secure attachment relationship during the year after birth. Toward the end of the first year, which is also the end of the sensorimotor period of Piaget, the mother's image is internalized by the infant. Therefore the appearance of an unknown person can evoke extreme anxiety in the infant (fear of strangers), because the infant compares the stranger with the internalized image of the mother.

Ainsworth et al. [13] postulated that the "strange situation procedure" can measure the extent to which the infant is attached to the mother at around the end of the first year of life. This procedure sets up a sequence of stressful situations for an infant, during which changes in the attachment behaviors to the mother or a stranger are observed. In these situations infants may demonstrate an insecure attachment relationship with the mother. For example, infants usually do not care about their mother's absence; if they did, anxiety caused by the absence of the mother would be diminished by the appearance of the mother. Those infants who have established a secure attachment relationship with the mother can leave the mother with a feeling of basic trust and attend to objects of interest.

Development of Interpersonal Social Relationships

Infants can develop a relationship with the father and siblings on the same basis as the secure attachment relationship with the mother. With acquisition of the ability to walk by themselves, infants can regulate their distance from the mother. Infants return quickly to the mother to restore their energy, to once again leave the mother to seek interests in the outer world—if the mother demonstrates emotional availability for the infant when the infant feels anxious about being too far from the mother. In short, students of Freud theorize that young infants start out by living as one unit with the mother, progress to live in an infant–mother world, and finally live in an infant–mother–father world.

With the increase in knowledge about infants' abilities, however, this theorizing seems to require correction. Here let me introduce the ideas of Mahler et al. [14]. She maintained that personality development in one's life cycle is the process of sparation–individuation. She named the first stage (first week after birth) as the normal autistic phase and the second stage (between 1 week and 36 months), which contains five phases, as the normal symbiotic phase, differentiation phase (5–9 months), practicing phase (9–14 months), rapprochment phase (14–24 months), and finally, "on the way to libidinal object constancy" phase (36 months). Apart from criticism [15] that the normal autistic phase would invite misunderstanding of the term "autistic," the infant of this age is well known to have a variety of abilities; hence it seems that the theory that a newborn does not recognize even the existence of the mother is defunct. These ideas might herald the ruin of the early contention that the newborn does not see or hear anything—that he or she is like a white paper on which many things can be impressed.

Position of "Infancy" in the Life Cycle

Continuity and Discontinuity in Development

It is often said that development, on one hand, is continuous and on the other hand discontinuous. Continuity, however, does not imply smooth or complete continuity; rather, it progressed with uneven speed throughout the life cycle. Moreover, discontinuity does not imply a simple quantitative change but, rather, changes in quality.

The issue of continuity–discontinuity during development is related to the prediction of later development based on that of the infant period. A high degree of continuity in one feature of development (e.g., intelligence, temperament, social ability, or mental disorder) means a high probability of correct prediction about the same feature during early development.

The feature considered most frequently is intelligence. A low intelligence level during infancy has been said to predict low intelligence during later life, even adulthood. This theorem has now been discarded owing to many criticisms that the methodology used to study the relation between early intelligence and that of a later period was inappropriate to make clear the subtle differences in intelligence for the two periods.

Continuity and Discontinuity in Neurological Development

It has been believed until recently that the development of the CNS can be accelerated when the fetus is brought outside the uterus because many incoming stimuli now reach the infant directly and so accelerate the development of the CNS. Much research has been done in which neurological development has been compared between infants born at term and those before term who are of the same postconceptional age. As a result, it is now almost established that CNS development is solely dependent on the postconceptional age and is independent of the length of intrauterine life. In other words, there is continuity in the development of the CNS between intrauterine and extrauterine life. Does this theory still hold true today, where new findings have been made available by the advances in modern clinical instrumentation?

De Vries et al. [16] have studied extensively the behaviors of the fetus using ultrasonography and have disclosed many hitherto unknown facts. They noted that the fetus has a repertoire of behaviors comparable to those of newborn infants—not only single behaviors but complex functions, such as state organization [17]. It can be said, therefore, that the fetus has developed almost the same degree of organized CNS activity at term as is found in the newborn. As a result we can see the continuity of development between the fetus and newborns.

On the other hand, many findings have pointed to discontinuity of CNS development between 2 and 3 months of age. For example, young infants demonstrate true antigravity posture and movements only after 2–3 months, and Wolff [18] has shown that the quality of sleep organization changes between 2 and 3 months of postnatal life.

Relation Between Infancy and Later Abnormal Development (Psychopathology)

Rutter [2] stressed the importance of the relation between infancy and later abnormal development in infant psychiatry and proposed the notation of "developmental psychopathology." Many researches in this vein have shown the most prevalent theme to be concerned with the relation between the quality of the infant–mother attachment relation and psychopathology during later development. Lewis et al. [19], for example, found that if boys build an insecure attachment relationship with their mother, they show some statisticaly significant signs of psychopathology at around 6 years of age. On the other hand, it cannot be said that every boy with an insecure attachment relationship develops psychopathology during later life. Therefore the most important question concerns a factor other than the attachment quality during infancy that may be the determinant for psychopathology during later life.

Chess and Thomas [20] summarized their long-term research on the longitudinal follow-up of different "temperaments," and their research can answer the posed question. They identified basically three types of temperament in the newborn—easy, difficult, and slow to warm up—and the rates for each type were 40%, 10%, and 15%, respectively. A total of 133 newborn infants were followed until they reached adolescence. It was found that the most prevalent psychopathology was found in children with a "difficult" temperament. The authors postulated that development is appropriate if the environment fits the individual temperament (goodness of fit), and that development is abnormal if the environment does not fit the temperament (poorness of fit) because a dissonance occurs between infant and mother. In other words, the combination of a difficult temperament in the infant and the conflict with the mother can produce psychopathology. Interestingly, it was also found that negative traditional life events, such as divorce of the parents or separation of the infant from a parent, are in themselves not risk factors for psychopathology.

Although new findings came out of this research, numerous questions were left to be answered. For example, what is the determining factor in the infants of difficult temperament who turned out to be normal in later life [21]?

Clinical Aspects of Infant Psychiatry

Developmental Checkup

The era is over when physical development alone was the most important area to be assessed. Today the holistic health of an individual has become the goal of the health care system. To obtain this goal, it is thought that mental development beginning in the infant and the establishment of a secure attachment relationship (on which mental development is based) are the most crucial issues [22]. Therefore it may be the most important task for infant psychiatrists to monitor mental development from the earliest time of life. In 1961 in Japan, health checkups at the age of 3 years were started, and in 1977 checkups at the age of 1.5 years were made routine; since then the rate of infants checked has been consistently higher than 85%. Although the health checkup did not include sufficient attention to the mental health of the infants, it is obvious that these health checkups have played an important role in the health care of infants in Japan.

The most important purpose of the health checkups is, needless to say, to predict the future ill condition at an early stage of life and to intervene and prevent such disease as early as possible. For this purpose repeated health checkups are needed to assess various aspects of development from an early stage of life. Most of the research on the predictability of the future from the early stage of life stresses the difficulty of this kind of prediction. Because it is evident that there is no single item with which we can predict a future mental condition, we should include as many items concerning mental health as possible. Various scales and assessment tools are currently used for the purpose of developmental diagnosis, and because many of them are "normality-dependent" tests we should keep in mind their limitations. Uzgiris and Hunt [23] proposed an assessment tool based on the ordinal scale of psychological development, which cancels out the drawback of the above-mentioned developmental test.

Japanese infant health care, which is mainly undertaken in Public Health Centers (PHCs), has been carried out with the limitation that only a diagnostic service is offered, unaccompanied by therapeutic intervention. Thus parents often face anxiety about their infant's condition without access to remedial intervention at the PHC. The most important point is that both the health checkup and any intervention required should be done in the same place (i.e., the PHC). Of course we shoud be aware of the principles on which these interventions are based, some of which have already been discussed; others are discussed below.

Prognosis of "High Risk" Infants

High risk infants are those whose proper development is disturbed for any reason from an early stage of life and who have a high likelihood of developing some disorder in the future. Clinical intervention for these infants is the most important task of infant psychiatry. There has been much research and many studies concerned with various kinds of high risk infant, such as those born to young parents (under 18 years old), infants born with congenital or hereditary disorders, those born to substance-abuse mothers (e.g., alcohol, cigarettes, drugs), preterm infants, small- or large-for-dates infants, and infants with brain damage due to birth trauma.

Touwen and Huisjes [24] concluded that the correlation between the neurological condition during the newborn period and that of young infants was high but low in schoolchildren. In other words, a less-than-optimal neurological condition in newborns (caused by perinatal troubles, for example) does not always lead to minor behavioral or neurologcial disorders. This statement can be easily understood when we take into account the modern theory of development. Sameroff [25] proposed the transactional model of development and contended that this model can explain the process of the establishment of disorders, such as an emotional disorder. He stated that the high risk condition does not always lead to production of a disorder because the former condition is of course affected by the intervention of the growing environment during the middle of the child's development. Even in present-day psychiatry, this model of development is not completely appreciated.

Currently, among the high risk infants those most thoroughly studied are the premature infants. Dunn [26] studied prospectively and longitudinally a large number of low-birth-weight (LBW) infants (Vancouver Study) and reported that minimal brain dysfunction (MBD) was found most prevalently (18%) among the LBW infants (only 6.5% among otherwise normally born infants.) However, inattentiveness was rarely found in these MBD children, and unexpectedly the learning disability was found more often among LBW infants.

Classification of Psychiatric Disorders of Infancy

It can be said that such psychiatric disorders or symptoms during infancy as the maternal deprivation syndrome, anaclitic depression, and infantile autism were studied fragmentarily before the introduction of infant psyciatry. Therefore the concept of infant psychiatry has merit in that those disorders or symptoms that have been considered randomly and not based on any unifying principle can now be combined in reasonable order in a cohesive whole. A classification of psychiatric disorders of infancy can be used as a tool for the arrangement.

There is only one classification system for infant psychiatry, as far as I can determine. It is the one devised by Call [27]. As he stated, it may be incomplete, but it offers the convenience of order in what was a chaotic field:

A. Healthy responses
　　1. Developmental crises (e.g., 8 months of anxiety)
　　2. Situational crises (e.g., birth of a sibling)
B. Developmental deviations
　　1. Deviation of maturational patterns without demonstrable brain deficit (e.g., environmental retardation)
　　2. Deviation of maturational patterns with a demonstrable brain defect (e.g., Down syndrome)
　　3. Deviation of maturational patterns due to bodily illness or defect, and with no CNS defect (e.g., muscular dystrophy)
C. Psychophysiological disorders (psychological factors affecting the physical condition)
D. Attachment disorders of infancy
　　1. Reactive attachment disorder of infancy
　　2. Attachment disorder, anaclitic type, major depression
　　3. Attachment disorder with food refusal
　　4. Attachment disorder, symbiotic type
　　　　a. Primary (child and primary parent remain in symbiotic union throughout the second year of life)
　　　　b. Secondary (child and parent regress to symbiotic union)
　　　　c. Focal (involving one bodily function)
　　　　d. Infantile sadomasochism
E. Posttraumatic stress disorder of infancy
F. Disturbed parent–child relationship

    1. Dyadic dissynchrony during infancy
    2. Power struggle around issues of control and discipline
    3. Parental exploitation of child
    4. Parental neglect of child
    5. Parental abuse of child
G. Behavioral disturbances of infancy
    1. Irritable infant
    2. Hyperactive child
    3. Attention deficit disorder
H. Communication disorders
    1. Developmental language disorder
    2. Delayed onset of speech
    3. Regression of language functions
    4. Syntactic problems
    5. Idiosyncratic speech (e.g., twin speech)
    6. Withholding of speech
    7. Retardation of symbolic language functioning
    8. Elective mutism
I. Other *DSM-III* diagnoses applicable to children less than age 3
    1. Eating disorders
        a. Pica
        b. Rumination
        c. Atypical eating disorder
    2. Sleep terror disorder
    3. Infantile autism
    4. Organic mental disorders
    5. Substance-induced organic mental disorders
    6. Fetal alcohol syndrome
    7. Organic brain syndrome
    8. Overanxiety disorder
    9. Gender identity disorder
    10. Psychological factors affecting physical disorder

Therapeutic Intervention and Treatment

Fraiberg et al. [28] described three modes of intervention or therapies for infant psychiatric problems: (1) short-term crisis intervention; (2) guidance for development; and (3) infant and parent psychotherapy. The first mode of intervention is needed when a sudden devastating change in the child-rearing condition occurs, and intervention is required to maintain infant mental health. In this case, because no problem in ego function or the child-rearing ability of the parents existed beforehand, the intervention can be short-term. The second type of intervention is required most often in clinical situations. For example, when an infant has had a chronic physical or emotional disease from early in life, the parents should be supported and the infant's develoment promoted and guided continuously throughout the intervention, which may be aimed at establishing a more secure infant–mother attachment relationship. In these cases the ego function of the parents is not always without problems; therefore a psychotherapeutic intervention for the parents may be needed so they can attain proper insight to their own problems. The last type of intervention is required when the parent has a psychiatric problem that affects the mental health of the infant. Intervention here is directed at having the parent gain insight into his or her own conflict and through such awareness relieve the infant of undue destructive involvement.

Viewed from another aspect, I believe there are two types of therapeutic intervention for psychiatric problems in infants. One is used for psychiatric problems that are already identified in the infant (this type is called an intervention of infancy in the narrow sense), for example, an intervention for intellectual retardation, interpersonal disturbances in autistic infants, or somatic symptoms of an attachment disorder. The other intervention is preventive and is used during a later period. An example is parental guidance to achieve enhanced development. More concretely, the following goals of parental guidance are mentioned.

1. To guide the parents to an appropriate understanding of the factors that inhibit the development of the infant. For example, information on the characteristics and long-term prognosis of congenital brain damage should be provided to the parents.

2. To guide the parents to acknowledge the possibility of being affected by the infant–mother relationship and being disturbed by the establishment of the infant–mother attachment relationship. The parents should be advised on how to avoid the risk of developing a disturbed attachment relationship. For example, early attachment behaviors, such as crying and eye contact, of the Down syndrome infant are poor in terms of both quantity and quality, which leads to decreased maternal responsiveness toward the infant and, further, to a disturbance of the attachment relationship between the two. Parents should be educated about this process and that a disturbance can cause developmental retardation of the infant. Parents should be encouraged to consciously have more frequent contact with the infant.

3. If the disturbing factors of infant development reside in the parents (e.g., the mother has a mental disease or conflicts), the desirable infant–mother relationship cannot be established. Even if the mother is aware of her psychiatric problem, she cannot do anything by herself to solve her problem. In such cases an intrafamilial condition in which the infant is situated at the center can be arranged and guides the family in a better direction.

4. In cases where there is no improvement after arranging a desirable infant-rearing situation in the family using the means outlined above, it may be necessary to elicit the cooperation of a social agency such as a Public Health Center, Child Guidance Clinic, and clinics or hospitals.

Closing Remarks

It should be kept in mind that infant psychiatry involves vast areas of endeavor; therefore it depends on other academic fields as well, such as developmental psychology, developmental neurology, gynecology, pediatrics, and human genetics. Infant psychiatry as a clinical science depends much on the future progress in basic medicine.

In the past we knew only the jargon of infant psychiatric problems, such as developmental retardation, infantile autism, abuse by parents, and so on. Now, however, we are equipped with an overall, comprehensive view of the subject, and, we can incorporate many concepts concerning infantile psychiatric problems in good order into this overall view. It is our future task.

References

1. Okonogi K (1987) An introduction to infant psychiatry (in Japanese). Hattatsu 32:1–42
2. Rutter M (1980) Scientific foundations of developmental psychiatry. Heinemann, London
3. Wolff PH (1966) The causes, controls and organization of behavior in the neonate. Psychological Issues Monograph Series 5. International Universities Press, New York
4. Prechtl HFR (1974) The behavioral states of the newborn infant [review]. Brain Res 76:185–212
5. Klaus M, Kennell J (1976) Maternal-infant bonding. Mosby, St. Louis
6. Papousek H (1961) Conditioned head rotation reflexes in infants in the first months of life. Act Paediatr Scand 50:565–573
7. Lipsitt LP (1986) Learning in infancy: cognitive development in babies. J Pediatr 109:172–182
8. Gibson JJ (1979) The ecological approach to visual perception. Houghton Mifflin, Boston
9. Thelen E, Kelso JAS, Vogel A (1987) Self-organizing systems and infant motor development. Dev Rev 7:39–65
10. Prechtl HFR (1984) Continuity and change in early neural development. In: Prechtl HFR (ed) Continuity of neural functions from prenatal to postnatal life. Blackwell, Oxford, pp 1–15
11. Ferrari F, Glosoli MV, Fontana G, Cavazutti GB (1983) Neurobehavioral comparison of low-risk preterm and fullterm infants at term conceptional age. Dev Med Child Neurol 25:450–458
12. Bowlby J (1969) Attachment and loss. Vol 1: Attachment. Basic Books, New York
13. Ainsworth MDS, Blehar MC, Waters E, Wall S (1978) Patterns of attachment: a psychological study of the strange situation. Erlbaum, Hillsdale, NJ
14. Mahler MS, Pine F, Bergman A (1975) The psychological birth of the human infant: symbiosis and individuation. Basic Books, New York
15. Klein M (1981) On Mahler's autistic and symbiotic phases: an expositon and evaluation. Psychoanal Contemp Thought 4:69–105
16. De Vries JIP, Visser GHA, Prechtl HFR (1984) Fetal motility in the first half of pregnancy. In: Prechtl HFR (ed) Continuity of neural functions from prenatal to postnatal life. Blackwell, Oxford, pp 46–64
17. Nijhuis JG, Martin CB Jr, Prechtl HFR (1984) Behavioural states of the human fetus. In: Prechtl HFR (ed) Continuity of neural functions from prenatal to postnatal life. Blackwell, Oxford, pp 65–78
18. Wolff PH (1984) Discontinuous changes in human wakefulness around the end of the second month of life: a developmental perspective. In: Prechtl HFR (ed) Continuity of neural functions from prenatal to postnatal life. Blackwell, Oxford, pp 144–158
19. Lewis M, Feiring C, McGuffog C, Jaskir J (1986) Predicting psychopathology in six-year-olds from early social relations. Child Dev 55:123–136
20. Chess, S, Thomas A (1987) Origins and evolution of behavior disorders: from infancy to early adult life. Harvard University Press, Cambridge, MA
21. Rutter M (1985) Resilience in the face of adversity: protective factors and resistance to psychiatric disorder. Br J Psychiatry 147:598–611
22. Nakayama K (1985) Principles in regular health check-ups. I. II (in Japanese). Pediatrics 26:1349–1356, 1809–1814
23. Uzgiris IC, Hunt JM (1975) Assessment in infancy: ordinal scales of psychological development. University of Illinois Press, Chicago
24. Touwen BCL, Huisjes HJ (1984) Obstetrics, neonatal neurology, and later outcome. Early Brain Damage 1:169–187
25. Sameroff AJ (1975) Early influences on development: fact or fancy? Merrill Palmer Q Behav Dev 21:267–294
26. Dunn HG (1986) Sequelae of low birth weight: the Vancouver study. Heinemann, London
27. Call JD (1984) Psychiatric syndromes in infancy. In: Call JD (ed) Basic handbook of child psychiatry, vol v. Basic Books, New York, pp 260–261
28. Fraiberg S, Shapiro V, Cherniss D (1983) Treatment modalities. In: Call JD, Galenson E, Tyson RL (eds) Frontiers of infant psychiatry, vol 1. Basic Books, New York, pp 56–73

Part 3

School Refusals

Nonattendance at School (School Phobia): Clinical Aspects and Psychopathology

Akira Nakane

Summary. This study suggests that nonattendance at school (school phobia) is not a clinical entity, a neurotic condition, but that it sometimes has definite features of various psychiatric disorders. After surveying the statistical, follow-up, and diagnostic approaches to this problem in Japan, we developed an overall picture of the psychopathology of school phobia in children and adolescents. Once students have been absent from school for any one of various reasons, they become afraid that classmates will ask them why they were absent. They develop specific "feelings of behindness," which means that there is a feeling of guilt by the student. Such feelings about not attending school develop into a chronic state, manifested by various neurotic disorders: separation anxiety disorder, panic disorder, obsessive-compulsive disorder, and social phobia. when these conditions are prolonged, the problems extend to family situations and finally to the state of the ego. The features of this stage are schizoid personality and borderline personality disorder. With the former, there is still a chance of readapting to school life, and such students can terminate their period of "school refusal." In some of the adolescents who have a school phobia, however, schizophrenic symptoms develop after some time.

Key words. School phobia—School refusal—Nonattendance at School—Psychopathology—Nosology

Background

The plight of childen with "school refusal," or school phobia, is a serious educational problem in Japan. As late as a decade ago, school refusal, as it is called in Japan, was considered a clinical disease entity—a neurotic disorder of children and adolescents. Most Japanese child psychiatrists now agreed that school refusal may be caused by various psychopathological conditions. School refusal has been a frequent topic of discussion at the Japanese Association for Child and Adolescent Psychiatry and Allied Professions (JACAPAP). At the first general meeting of JACAPAP in 1960, Sumi and

Division of Child and Adolescent Psychiatry, Tokyo Metropolitan Umegaoka Hospital, 6-37-10 Matsubara, Setagaya-Ku, Tokyo 156, Japan her colleagues and Nareta gave presentations on this subject based on the separation anxiety theory. Earlier, Takagi et al. [1] had noted the problem of children who do not attend school and had conducted a survey of schools in Kyoto. Takagi [2] attempted to divide the development of school phobia into three stages, each expressed through a characteristic clinical picture: (1) hypochondriacal stage; (2) agressive stage; and (3) seclusive stage. Takagi et al. [3] later stated that these stages were typical but that not all school phobics progress through them. Takagi refuted the separation anxiety theory of school phobia. This opinion, though initially controversial, then had been widely accepted in Japan at that time, and stands in marked contrast to the classification in the *Diagnostic and Statistical Manual 3rd Edition* (*DSM-III*), which treats school phobia as a separation anxiety disorder. As times and the society have changed, more of these students have come to act violently toward their mothers, and there is little evidence of the third, seclusive, stage.

Background Factors

Furukawa et al. [4] studied the frequency of "school haters," another name for school-phobic students, at public junior high schools in Tokyo from 1951 to 1978. A peak number of these students occurred between 1963 and 1966, followed by the lowest incidence in 1972; the incidence rose gradually thereafter. The number of school-phobic children differed by region, with commercial areas and new residential areas showing especially high rates. Furukawa et al. [4] suggested that school refusal was linked to socioeconomic conditions. They noted that factors affecting the incidence were as follows: (1) population density and personal economic factors; (2) cultural factors, such as the level of domestic stability, the level of neighborhood security, the amount of information available in homes, and educational standards; and (3) the rate of increase in number of households and in population.

Hishiyama et al. [5] conducted similar surveys throughout Japan and found regional differences in the incidence of school refusal between 1967 and 1978. The national mean rate decreased from 1972 to 1976, as did the rate for Tokyo. After 1976 the rates gradually increased.

Wakabayashi et al. [6] pointed out that statistics from the Department of Psychiatry at Nagoya University showed the lowest incidence of school refusal for the years 1972 and 1973. Before that date more male than female school phobics were treated, but the number of girls with this problem increased, and there has been no difference in the incidence rates of the genders since 1972. This shift in gender difference (increasing number of female school refusers) was paralleled by another shift in gender difference: the increased rate of girls entering senior high schools, junior colleges, and universities.

Honjo et al. [7] continued to collect data until 1984 and then compared the data of 1972–1974 with those of 1982–1984. The number of school-phobic subjects under age 13 at first contact with psychiatric services decreased during this period, whereas the number of those above age 13 increased markedly. Accompanying school refusal were such somatic symptoms as headaches, stomachaches, and fevers; violence toward the mother; and increasingly poorer school records. The number of female patients decreased during this period, contradicting the conclusion of Wakabayashi et al. that the increasing incidence of school refusal among girls and the increased number of girls entering upper-level schools were linked.

The data from these four studies show that school refusal is based on complex social factors and not on personal conflicts between mother and child alone. In 1993 the "school haters" in Japan numbered 14,763 in primary school and 59,993 in junior high school. These figures, which constituted 0.17% and 1.24% of the school populations, respectively, increased 0.02% and 0.08%, respectively, from 1992 [8].

Follow-up Surveys

Among follow-up surveys, the most significant are the long-term studies that have investigated social adaptability. Such surveys have extended 10 years from the subjects' first contact with psychiatric services, and the mean age of the subjects at outcome is 20 years or more.

Fukuma et al. [9] conducted a long-term follow-up study in Shimane Prefecture and found that 68.5% of school refusers at the junior high school level entered senior high school, compared to 83.9% the overall student population. The rate of school refusers in Japan who entered universities or junior colleges was 48.8%, whereas only 32.5% of high school students in the prefecture entered. The authors also found that 5 of 92 students (5.4%) suffered from schizophrenia after 10 years.

Umezawa [10] surveyed the prognoses of 40 school refusers who received residential treatment at Shimane Prefecture Koryo Hospital, which has a psychiatric ward with in-hospital classes for children and adolescents. Among those who were in the second to fourth years of the follow-up surveys, 31.6% were rated as poorly adjusted. As the duration of the follow-up period increased, however, fewer subjects were scored as maladjusted. Among those in the eighth to twelfth years of the follow-up, 1 of 12 (8.3%) was regarded as poorly adjusted. During the first year after discharge from the hospital 18 of 40 failed to attend school or to hold a job; during the second year this number was reduced to 13; and at the end of the survey 10 of the original 40 were not attending school or holding a job. This study indicates that the findings change according to the length of follow-up. In addition, those admitted to the hospital within 3 months from the beginning of their not attending school showed more favorable adjustment than those admitted after a longer interval. The mean time between onset of symptoms and admission among the well adjusted was 12.1 months, whereas among the poorly adjusted it was 20.5 months.

Ohtaka et al. [11] analyzed 40 long-term school refuses in the Department of Psychiatry in Nagoya University; 47% showed good social adaptation (group 1), 18% had problems but adapted somehow (group 2), and 35% evinced chronic problems in their social lives (group 3). Those in group 1 decided by themselves whether to enter university or technical school, start a part-time job, or obtain licenses or qualifications. In group 2, poor sociability and seclusiveness persisted, and many of these subjects dropped out after entering upper-level schools. Patients in group 3 continued to refuse schooling either by leaving the school or remaining absent for long periods; most were still receiving psychiatric treatment. These data indicate that the patient's prognosis is related to how closely he or she remains in contact with a school. Most of those who had a more successful recovery went to high school at night or met the qualifications for college admission that allowed them to end their school refusal, thereby readapting to normal life.

Nosological Aspects

It was previously thought that school refusal is a neurotic disorder, a unique clinical entity. It is now recognized, however, that subjects with neurotic symptomatology often show schizophrenic symptoms.

Yamamoto [12], in an early study, divided those with school phobia into two groups. The first, "core," group shows school phobia alone, lacking other neurotic symptoms. The second, "peripheral," group has various neurotic symptoms or features that suggest schizophrenia. The author suggested, however, that these two groups have the same disturbance—they cannot cope with their situation in school.

Minakawa et al. [13] sent questionnaires to researchers and clinicians in psychiatry throughout Japan asking if school refusal should be treated as an independent clinical entity. The responses were evenly divided: 47% of the responders believed that school refusal is an independent clinical entity, whereas the others did not. Of those who thought it an independent clinical entity, 74% believed it should remain in a diagnostic category that considers it a syndrome or clinical state. Later Yamazaki et al. [14] reported on two such subjects, one a typical and the other an atypical school phobic. These authors then sent these case reports to the same researchers and clinicians in Minakawa et al.'s study, asking them to diagnose the two cases according to the criteria in the *DSM-III*, ICD-10, and traditional Japanese classifications. For the typical case, 71% of psychiatrists diagnosed it as school refusal, but their *DSM-III* and ICD-10 (Draft) diagnoses included a wide range of neuroses. In contrast, 97% of psychiatrists denied that the atypical case constituted school refusal, and its diagnoses varied widely, such as schizophrenia, conduct disorder, and borderline personality disorder.

Yamazaki et al. [15] also asked two psychiatrists at the same school to diagnose school-phobic patients (after written consent was obtained from both patients and their parents), and the results were then compared. This trial was conducted at three hospitals: Tokai University Hospital, Keio University Hospital, and Tokyo Metropolitan Umegaoka Hospital. Twenty-eight patients from these three hospitals were examined to determine if the diagnosis was school refusal according to traditional diagnostic criteria. In this study, Yamazaki et al. [15] used two diagnostic criteria for school refusal: Criterion A focused on the mental state specific to school-phobic adolescents according to the criteria of Berg [16]; criterion B was a simplified form of criterion A. The results indicated that there was no significant difference between the cases diagnosed as school refusal and those not dignosed as school refusal according to both criteria A and criteria B. In addition, there was good agreement between the two psychiatrists when the cases were diagnosed as school refusal according to traditional diagnostic criteria; but when they were dignosed by ICD-10 criteria, the diagnoses by the two psychiatrists were quite different, being distributed in ICD-10 diagnostic categories F4 and F5. We have concluded therefore that school refusal is not an independent, unique syndrome, and that the reasons for these children and adolescents not attending school stemmed from various psychiatric conditions.

From this viewpoint, Nakane et al. [17] studied 87 inpatients (52 boys, 35 girls) admitted to Tokyo Metropolitan Umegaoka Hospital from January 1986 to December 1989 with a diagnosis of school refusal or similar condition. The physicians then reexamined their diagnoses at 1.5 to 3.0 years after admission. In this study we found 22 schizophrenics among the 87 subjects (i.e., 25% of all patients: 15 boys, 29%; 7 girls,

Table 1. Nosological diagnoses 13–16 months after admission.

Diagnosis	Male (no.)	Female (no.)	Total no.	%
Schizophrenia	15	7	22	25.3
Adjustment disorder	12	4	16	18.4
Depressive disorder	3	10	13	14.9
Borderline personality disorder	5	6	11	12.6
Obsessive-compulsive disorder	3	0	3	3.5
Other anxiety disorders	4	6	10	11.5
Others[a]	10	2	12	13.8
Total	52	35	87	100.0

From [17], with permission.

[a]Hyperkinetic disorder, mental retardation, borderline intelligence, and others.

20%) (Table 1). In our hospital patients are admitted to adolescent wards because of nonattendance at school only if they have severe behavioral problems with profound psychopathology. It should be noted that 20%–30% of the patients who are nonattenders at school may become schizophrenic. Moreover some outpatients with long absences from school develop schizophrenic symptoms several years later, although the clinical features are the same as these seen with neurotic school phobia.

Psychopathology

In 1988 we reported our residential treatment and suggested that there is a specific maladjustment that develops into a chronic state in patients who did not attend school [18].

It should be stressed that school refusal does not mean simply a long period of absence; it is an abnormal process wherein the prolonged absence from school leads to social dysfunction. The key factor is not why the child *refuses* to go to school, but why he or she *cannot*. We believe this process begins at the time of the original absence. As the period of absence from school lengthens, daily life at home deteriorates and acting out frequently occurs.

Difficulties Attending School Due to Maladjustment

When something goes wrong in the classroom, some students are unable to cope with the circumstance, and they develop maladjustment. Each morning thereafter the child becomes tense before going to school, and psychosomatic symptoms occur, thereby preventing him or her from attending school. At this point the students believe themselves that they are ill, so they do not become anxious. Soon after, though, their parents (or caretakers) force them to go to school, and the subjects suffer intense self-reproach because they are then conscious of having stayed away from school without being ill ("feelings of behindness" in Japan, meaning "I feel some guilt behind me"). This feeling of behindness is the main mechanism responsible for prolonging nonattendance at school in Japan. They avoid leaving their house for fear of meeting someone in the neighborhood or classmates, even though they may find it agonizing to stay home with nothing to do. Sooner or later they become dysphoric.

Intrafamilial Maladjustment Caused by Prolonged Absence from School

To relieve the tension that occurs before going to school, these students decide to abandon every effort to attend school for a while. Usually adolescents do not want to hear or be asked about themselves, especially when they have done something wrong. Many children and adolescents who are school phobics rebel against the pressure exerted by their parents to go to school and seclude themselves in their own rooms or act aggressively toward their mothers. Some adolescents become mute to the father or attack their siblings. There is nowhere at home where they behave properly. We named this condition intrafamilial maladaptation, because the maladjustment increases, moving from the school environment to include the family. This psychological process is still reversible at this stage, as some students can overcome these situations and attend school regularly.

Pan-maladjustment Caused by Repeated Failure of Attempts to Go to School

Having failed attempts to attend school on several occasions, adolescents suffer painful damage to their minds. These young people then often act out, justifying this behavior to themselves or reproaching others for not meeting their needs. They spend all their time without trying to finds solution. Usually a change in environment, such as admission to an adolescent ward, temporarily alleviates the problem. Even if they return to school, a crisis occurs sooner or later. They often fail to continue to attend classes because of their inability to endure strain and stressful events. This situation damages their self-image, and they soon develop strong feelings of low self-esteem because they are not completing the course of study in school. We named this condition pan-maladjustment. It infers maladjustment in school, in the neighborhood, among the family, and in their own mind. Although avenues for normal social life are still available, many patients develop a personality disorder. These difficult patients may be diagnosed as having a borderline personality disorder based on their severe acting out, depression, and other behaviors.

Temporary Adjustment to Society and End of School Refusal

As they grow older these students try to adapt to society on their own. They start to attend high school evening classes, prepare themselves to take a qualification examination for college entrance, or choose correspondence school courses in attempts to reenter society. If they have grown internally they can overcome their feelings of low self-esteem and learn to overcome difficult situations. Althought this stage may not occur until they reach 18 years of age, they probably can now end their long-term school refusal.

In primary school students, the "feeling of behindness" occurs only in relation to classmates and does not damage their self-esteem as is seen in adolescents. They avoid school only to avoid the judgment of their peers and teachers. They stay home close to their mothers. Once they decide to go back to school, however, they achieve the transition with relative ease.

New Directions

Recently, the attitudes surrounding school refusal have changed in Japan. The school now allows the absence of school-phobic students, and pressure to force them to attend school by parents and teachers is reduced. Accordingly, child psychiatrists believe that aggressive behavior and seclusion occur less often. We suggest here a diagnostic framework for considering school refusal.

School refusal begins as an adjustment disorder. In some students chronic fatigue is the first symptom, and they cannot wake up in morning. Miike and Tomoda [19] conducted a systematic examination of central nervous system (CNS) functions and pointed out that weakened activity of information processes caused by brain function fatigue results in a blocking their studying; hence they feel unable to go to school. Other students have somatic complaints just before they are to leave for school. This condition resembles "somatoform autonomic dysfunction." Some senior high school adolescents report depressive moods that progress to a persistent mood disorder (dysthymia).

After "feelings of behindness" are present, many nonattending students exhibit anxiety. If there is excessive anxiety in young students, they may not be able to leave their mothers and position their bodies near the mother whenever awake and even during sleep (separation anxiety disorder). In other cases, it manifests as a violent attack of intense anxiety, otherwise known as panic disorder [20]. Some students remain peaceful so long as they are in their house; however, when they step out the door or walk around and come near the school building they experience panic (agoraphobia). Obsessive-compulsive disorder is a common complication as well. The most frequent form of a school-phobia reaction is the inability to enter places where young people or students gather (social phobia).

Over long periods of nonattendance at school, various psychopathological states develop; among them are such chronic states as schizoid personality and borderline personality disorder. With the former condition patients are able to decide to return to school life and can end the long process of school refusal. The latter condition, borderline personality disorder, continues when the adolescents become adults. Even if they work within the society, some act out; and an aggressive outburst may occur even after many years. Unfortunately, some adolescents with nonattendance at school develop schizophrenic symptoms.

References

1. Takagi R, Kawabata T, Tamura S, et al (1959) Psychiatric survey of long absentees from obligation of school attendance (in Japanese). Clin Psychiatry 1:403–409
2. Takagi R (1963) Mental mechanism of school phobia and its prevention. Acta Paedopsychiatr 30:135–140
3. Takagi R, Kawabata T, Fujisawa A, Kato N (1965) Nuclear type of school phobia. 1. Symptom formation (in Japanese with English abstract). Jpn J Child Psychiatry 6:157–165
4. Furukawa, H, Hishiyama Y (1980) A statistical study of the refusal to attend school. 1. Social factors and the change in the incidence rate in Tokyo (in Japanese with English abstract). Jpn J Child Adolesc Psychiatry 21:300–309
5. Hishiyama Y, Furukawa H (1982) A statistical study of the refusal to attend school. 2. Socical factors and the change in the incidence rate in Japan (in Japanese with English abstract). Jpn J Child Adolesc Psychiatry 23:183–191

6. Wakabayashi S, Kaneko T, Saburi M, et al (1982) The relationship between school refusal and social conditions in Japan (in Japanese with English abstract). Jpn J Child Adolesc Psychiatry 23:160–180

7. Honjo S, Kaneko T, Wakabayashi S, et al (1987) The actual conditions of patients who refuse to go to school: change from 1972–74 to 1982–84 (in Japanese with English abstract). Jpn J Child Adolesc Psychiatry 20:33–35

8. Ministry of Education (1994) Report of a survey of fundamental school education problems (in Japanese). Yomiuri Shimbun 1994 August 13

9. Fukuma H, Inoue E, Namine T, et al (1980) Long-term follow-up of school phobic children and adolescents (in Japanese). Clin Psychiatry 22:401–408

10. Umezawa Y (1984) School refusal and modern society, from the follow-up study of residential treatment in Japan (in Japanese). Jpn J Child Adolesc Psychiatry 25:85–89

11. Ohtaka K, Wakabayashi S, Enomoto K, et al (1986) A long-term follow-up study of school refusal children (in Japanese with English abstract). Jpn J Child Adolesc Psychiatry 27:213–219

12. Yamamoto Y (1964) Über die Pathogenese der sogenanten Schulphobie (in Japanese with German abstract). Psychiatr Neurol Jpn 66:558–583 (abstract on pp 38–39)

13. Minakawa K, Nakane A, Miyake Y, et al (1989) Inquiry on clinical diagnosis of school refusal. Jpn J Psychiatry Neurol 43:311

14. Yamazaki K, Kurita H, Minakawa K, et al (1989) Study of diagnostic classification of child and adolescent psychiatric disorders. 2. Report of a national research project concerning the genesis of and treatment for child and adolescent psychiatric disorders 1988 (in Japanese). National Center of Psychiatry and Neurology, pp 79–92

15. Yamazaki K, Kurita H, Minakawa K, et al (1990) Study of diagnostic classification of child and adolescent psychiatric disorders. 3. Report of a national research project concerning the genesis of and treatment for child and adolescent psychiatric disorders 1989 (in Japanese). National Center of Psychiatry and Neurology, pp 75–87

16. Berg I (1980) School refusal in early adolescence. In: Hersov L, Berg I (eds) Out of school: modern perspective in truancy and school refusal. Wiley New York, pp 231–249

17. Nakane A, Kato H, Hara K, et al (1991) School refusal, its relation to schizophrenia and mood disorders (in Japanese). Jpn J Psychiatr Treat 6:1173–1179

18. Nakane A (1990) School refusal: psychopathology and natural history. In: Chiland C, Young G (eds) Why children reject school: view from seven countries. Yale University Press, New Haven, pp 62–72

19. Miike T, Tomoda A (1994) Death by overwork in school: what happened in the body in the state of non-attending school children (in Japanese). Shindan To Chiryo Sha, Tokyo

20. Deshimaru M, Ishizuka K, Tsuji Y, Miyakawa T (1994) Panic disorder in puberal cases with school refusal (in Japanese). Clin Psychiatry 35:241–248

School Refusal and Family Pathology: Individualized and Multifaceted Approach

Kayoko Murase

Summary. Thirty cases of school refusal that ended with clear results over a 10-year period are reviewed. The results showed that an individualized, multifaceted approach is clinically effective for treating school nonattendance. School refusal is not a clinical entity but a phenomenon complicated by many factors, such as (1) the problems of the child, (2) the family configuration, and (3) social factors including the school situation. For effective treatment, it is essential to understand what the child wants to accomplish by not going to school and to comprehend not only the problems of the child but also the structures of the family, school, and community. The principles of our therapy are (1) to determine the potential of the client; (2) not to persuade the child to go back to school prematurely but to encourage him or her at the appropriate time when it would be effective; (3) to wait until the child develops some maturity; and (4) to find hobbies or activities in which the child is interested and that can be shared with the therapist. We call these activities "windows or channels of the heart." Even the most seclusive clients have the potential to open themselves to and maintain contact with the outer world through specific interests. By sharing these activities, we can establish and maintain the therapeutic relationship and help such children grow psychologically and socially. The two final principles of our therapy program are (5) to obtain cooperation from the family by explaining the situation of the client and being supportive of them; and (6) to maintain contact with the school with the consent of the client.

Key Words. School refusal—Multifaceted approach—Therapist tutor—Windows or channels of the heart—Life experience group

Introduction

In a modern high-technology society, there is a strong tendency to value people only by their productive efficiency. In such a society, a number of children do not feel that they are accepted as they are, and their number is increasing.

Understanding school refusal requires consideration of several elements: (1) factors having to do with the child (personality, infantile conflicts, trauma during early childhood, psychological conflicts in the present situation, identity crisis during ado-

School of Human Studies, Taisho University, 3-20-1 Nishi-Sugamo, Toshima-ku, Tokyo 170, Japan
Mailing address: 6-22-4 Hongomagome, Bunkyo-ku, Tokyo 113, Japan

72

lescence) [1]; (2) factors in the family (emotionally inadequate family relationships, role confusion and dysfunction in the family, symbiotic relationship between parent and child, unfulfilled object relations) [2, 3]; (3) social factors (for example, children may get no individualized attention at school, even though individuality is valued in principle, because group-oriented preparation for entrance exams is more efficient and is stressed).

School refusal is not a clinical entity; it is a syndrome with diverse causes. In recent years, there are increasing numbers of cases of school refusal with jeopardized personality development manifested by poor verbal expression, extreme acting-out behaviors, and somatic complaints.

Successful therapy depends largely on how accurately one understands (1) what a child is trying to achieve through school refusal, (2) the nature of the problems of the child, (3) the specific structures of the family, school, and community surrounding the child. In addition to giving psychological help to the child and parents, the therapist must have a therapeutic perspective that determines when, where, and by whom help can be given, the specific aspects of the problem that must be addressed, and how the therapy can be organized. To do so, the therapist must grasp the whole picture surrounding the child. This approach comprises our individualized, multifaceted program [4].

When facing this therapeutic challenge, the therapist must consider several principles simultaneously. The first priority is to look for the potential strengths of the child. At the same time, encouraging the child to go back to school too soon is avoided, waiting for the appropriate time, while observing and fostering inner maturity. To achieve these goals, it is essential to nourish the therapeutic alliance by establishing a "windows of the heart"[1] [5], that is, finding and nurturing the child's routines and hobbies that can be shared with others and can become sources of a mutual "language" with the therapist.

Clinical Cases

The syndrome of school refusal commonly coexists with several disorders. The cases outlined below do not include patients who were diagnosed during the evaluation as suffering from schizophrenia, depression, deliquency, or obvious truancy. Those unable to attend school because of acute obsessive symptoms were diagnosed as having obsessive-compulsive neurosis and were omitted from the study. Also not included are the clients whose parents came for advice because they felt uneasy or dubious about the treatment their children were receiving elsewhere. Supportive measures were taken with these parents, but no direct contact was made with the children.

Description of Cases

The characteristics of each case and the components of treatment are shown in Table 1. Family structure and outcome are also noted. The outcome was rated as good, moderate, or poor. As all the clients went back to school, the main criteria of the

---

[1] This metaphorical expression symbolizes the medium through which the relationship between therapist and client can sprout and through which the client can learn new, more appropriate ways to relate to other people or things.

Table 1. Characteristics of clinical cases and their treatment.

Case no.	Sex	Age[a]	Concomitant symptoms	Violence[b]	Harshly teased[c]	Family structure[d]	Father < mother[e]	Conflict between generations, brothers and sisters[f]	Medical treatment[g]	Provisional termination[h] (months)	Style of therapy[i]	Therapeutic tutor	Life experience group	Contact with school	Window of the heart	Outcome
1	F	7 (3)	Taciturn	○●	○	(diagram)	Yes		○↕	4	3, 6			Yes	Squiggle technique riddles w/drawings, making lunch together	Poor
2	M	7 (3)	Headaches, stomachaches			(diagram)		○	↕	3	2				Appealing to his mother w/needs for affection	Good
3	F	7 (4)	Headaches, continuous			(diagram)		●	↕	2	3				Fantasy story writing, smoking	Good
4	M	8 (2)	Pain all over body		●	(diagram)		●	↕	3	2			Yes	Jogging w/his mother	Good
5	F	10 (2)	Anorexia nervosa, taking mother's money			(diagram)	Yes	●	↕	1	3, 6			Yes	Carrying as an amulet a slip of paper with therapist's address and phone number	Good
6	F	11 (2)	Taciturn at certain times		○	(diagram)			#↕	2	3, 4, 5			Yes	Squiggle technique, sand play technique, crafts	Good
7	F	11(2)	Stomachaches, anorexia nervosa		●	(diagram)		●	↕	3	4				Animals, sports, mischievous tricks	Good

No.	Sex	Age (onset)	Symptoms			Pedigree									Interests	Outcome
8	F	12 (since age 8)	Headaches, stomachaches		○	(pedigree)	Yes	●	↑ # ↕	26	3, 4, 5	Yes	Yes	Yes	Cartoons, story making	Good
9	M	13 (since age 4)	Stomachaches	●○	○	(pedigree)	Yes	●		22	3,6	Yes		Yes	Vehicle play, fishing, raising animals, eating together	Good
10	M	13 (12)	Headaches, nausea	●○	○	(pedigree)	Yes	○	#	12	3, 4, 5	Yes		Yes	Poem and novel writing, drawing	Good
11	F	12 (5)	Taciturn at certain times		○	(pedigree)	Yes	●		18	3, 4, 5		Yes	Yes	Raising a weed (self image), raising animals, sports, cartoons	Good
12	M	13 (4)	Taciturn at certain times, asthma		○	(pedigree)	Yes		↑ ↕	18	3, 4, 5	Yes	Yes	Yes	Raising animals, sand play techniques, cooking	Good
13	F	13 (since age 5)	Packing knapsack to leave home			(pedigree)	Yes			5	3		Yes	Yes	Drawing, raising animals	Good
14	F	13 (3)	Stomachaches		○	(pedigree)	Yes			3	3, 4	Yes	Yes	Yes	Playing an electric organ, rock music, animals	Good
15	M	13 (5)	Headaches, kidney ailment		●	(pedigree)	Yes	●	↑ ↕	3	3			Yes	Drawing, making personal computer games	Good
16	F	14 (since age 11)	Scrupulous about her appearance		○	(pedigree)				2	3, 4, 5			Yes	Table tennis, cooking, learning to do household chores for ill mother	Good
17	M	14	Running away, stomachaches	●○	○	(pedigree)				17	3, 4, 5			Yes	Writing poems, crafts, sewing	Good

Table 1. Continued.

Case no.	Sex	Age[a]	Concomitant symptoms	Violence[b]	Harshly teased[c]	Family structure[d]	Father < mother[e]	Conflict between generations, brothers and sisters[f]	Medical treatment[g]	Provisional termination[h] (months)	Style of therapy[i]	Therapeutic tutor	Life experience group	Contact with school	Window of the heart	Outcome
18	F	14 (8)	Fever			(genogram)	Yes	○		8	3, 4, 5			Yes	Animals, stuffed animals, secret telephone calls, toll calls, lunch	Good
19	F	14 (3)	Fever, headaches		●	(genogram)	Yes	○	○	3	3, 4	Yes			Table tennis	Good
20	M	14 (2)			○	(genogram)	Yes	●		2	2				Taking relief in the change in his mother	Moderate
21	F	15 (4)	Allergic asthma, anorexia nervosa	○ ●	○	(genogram)	Yes		○↕	8	3	Yes	Yes	Yes	Drawing, hugging filthy dogs, tennis, playing piano	Good
22	F	15 (since age 11)	Pain all over body		○	(genogram)	Yes	●	○↕	9	3, 6	Yes	Yes	Yes	Cooking, reading, table tennis	Good
23	M	15 (3)	Headaches		○	(genogram)	Dead			3	3	Yes		Yes	Reading philosophy and literature, rock music	Good
24	M	16 (9)	Various mental complaints	○		(genogram)	Yes		○	2	2				Father's understanding the client's feelings, secret telephone calls	Good
25	M	16 (3)	Anorexia nervosa	○		(genogram)	Yes	●		5	2	Yes		Yes	Matters concerning motorcycles	Moderate

No.	Sex	Age (months)[a]	Presenting problem	Violence[b]	Harsh teasing[c]	Family[d][e]	Generations / siblings[f]	Treatments[g]	Period[h]	Continued for years[a]	Interests / activities[i]	Outcome
26	M	16 (3)	Various mental complaints	○	Yes	○	○ ●	7	3		Subject of religion	Good
27	F	16 (3)	Shoplifting with friends	○	Yes	○		6	3	Yes	Chinese, subjects on Chinese culture	Good
28	F	16 (3)	Headaches	○		○	○ ↑	1	4, 5	Yes	Sand play techniques, movies, rock music	Good
29	M	15 (3)	Headaches		Yes		○	3	2		Classical music, seeing society through a part-time job	Good
30	M	19 (7)	Minimal brain dysfunction	○ ●		●	○ ↑	5	3, 4, 6	Yes	Table tennis, badminton, painting	Poor

a The age at which the client presented; the number in parentheses represents months passed since symptoms began. In some cases (where marked) symptoms have continued for years.

b Violence before consultation ○; after consultation ●.

c Especially harsh teasing ●.

d □, male; ○, female; ‖, marriage; —, parent–child; ■ or ●, client.

e Father < mother means weak family participation of father; Dead = father dead.

f Relationship between generations (grandparents, aunts, and uncles) clearly affecting the family symptoms ○; conflicts between brothers and sisters ●.

g Those treatments before consultation ○; those received in the Department of Psychiatry ↑; Department of Internal Medicine #; elsewhere ↑.

h Period it took to return to school or to initiate a new way of life.

i Style of therapy and last five columns are explained in greater detail in the text.

outcome rating were personality development and social adaptation. The explanation of each category is indicated in the footnotes to the table; the numbers shown for "style of therapy" refer to the therapeutic modalities described in the following list.

1. Therapist → child   therapist for child only
2. Therapist → parent   therapist for parent only
3. Therapist ↗ child   therapist for child and parent
   ↘ parent
4. Therapist → child   different therapists for parent and child
   Therapist → parent
5. Therapist ⇉ child   therapists for parent and child alternate occasionally
   Therapist ⇉ parent
6. Therapist ⤳ child   joint therapist(s) for parent and child
   (Therapist) → parent

We combine these modalities when it is necessary.

The "therapeutic tutor" [6] column indicates whether the therapeutic approach made use of a college or graduate student hired to help the child catch up on schoolwork and to supplement the child's play and activities in the neighborhood. The therapeutic tutor acts in a domain between that of a therapist and a usual home tutor who helps only with academic learning.

The term "life experience group" refers to a type of environmental therapy [7], or life experience therapy. Recently, we have seen many clients whose core personality is vague and for whom experience does not make sense. This "core" is supposed to develop at an early stage of life, and so it is useful to return to the period when the developmental disorder began and help the child grow again. To do it we must determine what can be done now and then find a way to realize this goal.

At the Taisho University Counseling Institute we establish a flexible therapeutic relationship, free from the therapeutic framework, although we fully understand the importance of the therapeutic structure and its restrictions. Time schedules and activities are selected according to the client's needs. The activities include having meals together, modifying the physical setting in the institute together, participating in sports or shopping, buying toys and tools for the institute based on a given plan and budget, and group study and learning through cooperative communication (for example, a young client telephones an older one with high scholastic ability who cannot leave home, asking for help with something he does not understand). What we call the "life experience group approach" is a component of our flexible methods.

"Contact with school" means that the therapist had direct contacts with the school the child had attended. The "Window of the heart" column shows the activities through which the client and therapist built their relationship and which helped clients change their ways so they could cope with other people, things, or themselves.

Case M: Individualized, Multifaceted Approach

There are two reasons I chose to describe case M in detail. First, it is a typical case that shows how the individualized, multifaceted approach works in the therapeutic process. Second, the client gave permission for the case to be published if it would help people who are suffering from a situation similar to his. Certain descriptions have been changed to protect the client's privacy.

Role of Therapist

Daily happenings and passing time may appear trivial in human growth and development but are in fact fundamental, which is also true for the process of therapy for school refusers. Not only the therapist but also the various elements around the client contribute to his or her healing and growth. Even silence in the interview session or the client's favorite activities that seem to be boring and repetitive are often a catalyst for growth, although it may be barely apparent.

If the therapeutic process is likened to a theatrical play, the therapist may be considered the scriptwriter and director, evaluating the client's problem, offering what the client needs, and being responsive and responsible during treatment. Alternatively, the client can be considered the stage itself and the therapist a *kuroko* (a stagehand in a kabuki play), in the sense that the therapist acts to help and watch over the people and matters on the stage. The therapist's role is to understand the client's position in relation to daily concerns and to the people around the client from a broad perspective, to maintain the relationship through the activities in which the client is interested, and to help the client to strengthen his or her ability to adjust at timely points.

The Encounter

The client, M (case 9 in Table 1), had been absent repeatedly from kindergarten and elementary school since age 4. After entering junior high school, he completely withdrew and began to lock the door of his room and eat alone. The family consists of his parents, both of whom hold professional jobs, a sister 5 years older than him, and the client.

When M was in seventh grade, his father came alone for a consultation. He listed M's faults and was somewhat reluctant to participate, saying that he and his wife are too busy for consultation. The therapist sent a postcard, "Landscape with a White Horse" by Kaii Higashiyama, asking M to come to the Institute to meet the therapist. (The tranquil picture conveys an image of traveling within the inner self and was sent with the therapist's hope of traveling with M in his inner world.)

M agreed to meet the therapist if she would come to his house. The therapist agreed to visit the client's home for several reasons: (1) because of the parents' reluctance for therapy; (2) in order to decide promptly if M's prolonged absence from school required medical treatment; (3) to make the most of the preliminary indication of the client's motivation to the therapy; and (4) to ask M to come to the Institute.

In the home, the living room was small and dark. The sliding door of the room was in tatters. Parents told the therapist that M's room was even worse, and that M had created all of the destruction. A fat, dirty M, who was 162 cm tall and weighed 78 kg, appeared and stared at the therapist. He sat leaning on the wall, stretched his legs in front of him and kicked the therapist's knee. He was defiant and rebellious. The parents, flustered, retreated to the kitchen.

After the therapist introduced herself, a fat dirty cat with no whiskers appeared and hopped onto her lap. Startled, M stared at the therapist. The therapist, petting the cat, asked if he liked cats. He said he did, and she continued, "So do I. Animals are honest, aren't they?"

"Yeah."

"Cats can't shave their own whiskers. You did it, didn't you?"

"Yeah."

They continued talking about cats, and the therapist eventually asked, "Why don't you come to therapy?" It prompted M to reply, "Yeah, I will." (M later reminisced, "I picked up the stray cat when I was in the third grade and still had a belief in people. I cared for the cat like it was a part of me. But as I gave up on people and felt miserable, I got mad at the cat. So, the cat was afraid of not just me but also any other people and hardly came out during the daytime. I was surprised when the cat hopped onto your lap because it stayed away from everyone.)

M began to come for therapy, though he was sometimes late or absent because of oversleeping. His parents dared to say, "We gave up on M," at that time. The school was also at a loss and did nothing. Considering those situations, the therapist set the following goals for treatment.

1. M was suspicious of everyone and everything and had lost his self-confidence. To give him more life experiences, the therapist would share the activities in which M was interested and then gradually expand them into the world outside.

2. His social relationships were awkward, although M wanted these relationships deep in his mind. A therapist tutor would be called in when M himself wanted one.

3. The family relationships were fragmented. M felt abandoned by his parents. It must have been one of the reasons that M clung to the house and had few experiences outside. One of the therapist's thoughts was that even a small change in M through therapy would bring the parents' hope back and reunite the family.

4. The therapist would keep in contact with the school and ask them to tell M periodically during the therapeutic process that they were waiting and there was a place for him in the school.

5. The parents were not cooperative because of their unpleasant experience with previous counselors. They feared that they would be accused of being the cause of M's problems. The therapist would listen to them without critical remarks, not talking about what should have been done but about what could be done now and help them to bring it to reality.

Emergence of M's Self-Expression and Communication Within the Family (Second Semester to Middle of Third Semester of Seventh Grade)

At first, M lived with day and night reversed and missed appointments or was late because of oversleeping; but gradually he came to therapy on time. He had suffered extreme loss of self-confidence, saying, "My knowledge is as poor as a fourth grader. I haven't played with friends ever since I could remember. Even my parents gave up on me and don't care. I have nothing to be proud of." Occasionally, however, the therapist had a glimpse of his competence. For example, when talking about foods he seemed to have elaborate tastes. Judging from his perceptive remarks about the contradictory attitudes of adults, his intelligence appeared to be above average and his sensitivity sophisticated. Without the love he wished for, however, he pretended indifference.

Hearing of his interest in trains, the therapist bought some related magazines, such as *Railway Journal*, to read with M, and they constructed elaborate models of trains with cardboard together that eventually became useful toys for small children in the playroom. Though claiming "I hate kids," he went to a model shop to buy the material. On the way he rode a bike for the first time in years, but his obesity made it awkward. He wanted to lose weight, so the therapist suggested sports and changes in his diet.

The therapist played table tennis with M. Because of his lack of fitness, M stumbled and fell down, but when he occasionally hit a great smash, he gave a big smile. At home he told his mother that the therapist was better at table tennis than he had expected and also quite good at throw and catch. This was the first time M had voluntarily spoken to his mother in years.

Moved by the slight change in M and appreciating the therapist doing sports with M, each parent took the initiative to come to consultation separately. However, they each criticized the other from their own one-sided view. The father claimed that the mother was stubborn and never repented or apologized. He warned the therapist not to be fooled by her. He described her as an able worker but a terrible housekeeper who devoted herself to her work and religion. It was she who ruined their home, from his point of view. The mother claimed that the father was vain, was often drunk, and looked at reality only from a distorted point of view. She said, "He was justly placed as a 'window-side worker' [an employee who is no longer considered to be competent to do important jobs] and remained psychologically dependent on his mother."

According to M, "Father is weak. He spends rashly just to show off and escapes into gambling and drinking. But Mother is so strong and stubborn that she is pushing him into drinking. Strong women ruin men. I have been mutilated by her for fourteen years."

The three of them thus insulted one another, and finally each challenged the therapist to try to convert the others into stable persons if she could. It was "therapy by commission."

At a session during this period, M mentioned a late-night Italian movie, "Sunflower"[1] he had seen. Coincidentally, his parents had also separately seen it in the theater, and each said, "I was deeply moved." For M, it was the first and last thing this couple ever agreed on. "This is one of the seven wonders of the world!" M exclaimed. The therapist responded, "They seemed to hate each other so much, but there is at least one thing they agree about. Maybe deep down inside they are looking for a tie they have lost, as in that movie." Surprised, M said, "What a way to think about it! You are different!" This episode seemed for the therapist to be a fragile thread that barely held together this awkward, stubborn, lonely family.

Beginning of Adaptation of and Acceptance of the Outer World
(Middle of Third Semester of Seventh Grade to the End of Eighth Grade)

The therapist and M reviewed his eating habits to help him lose weight, which revealed the family's unbalanced diet, which included much junk food. In addition, although M was intelligent enough to criticize others with acute and touching expressions, he lacked common sense about daily life because he had been left alone at home for a long time. Having talked about learning practical skills of daily life during therapy, M began to help with household chores, such as preparing dinner or a hot bath. This help gave his mother some relief; she had been experiencing stressful tension for a long time, doing all the housework by herself as well as earning money to help support the household.

---

[1] The movie depicts a war-related tragedy. During World War II a wife hears that her husband died in the Soviet Union, but she cannot believe it and visits the country after the war. There she finds out that her husband survived a near-fatal injury and married the woman who saved his life. Having seen their happy home, she goes back to Italy feeling disconsolate. The husband visits her in Italy with a gift of a fur coat, but they cannot restore the past.

M had had no friends since childhood and was reluctant to join in group activities, saying he was frightened by people other than the therapist. M had never been on a family vacation as far as he remembered, so during the summer holiday the therapist invited him to her home. He was reluctant but came to visit mainly because of a chance to ride trains on the way. The therapist took M and her child to a fishing pond. Even though it was not a good day for fishing, rainy and windy, M caught many fish, one after another, like a miracle. The child of the therapist exclaimed, "You are a fishing genius, aren't you!"

M thought, "This kid means it. His words are spontaneous. Adults' words are always thought out and planned, no matter how nice they are." After this occasion, M went fishing with his father, whom he had despised. He remarked; "Sitting silently with fishing rods, we seemed to understand each other's feelings, but it might have been an illusion." It must have been subtle communication.

The mother said grimly, "M said to me, 'Mrs. Murase is a working woman, but she cooked and treated me with nice things to eat. Work isn't an excuse.' I've been working hard outside home, determined not to lose my opportunities." She then began to pay more attention to her home life, and the change was evident in M's clothes being kept clean.

Because M complained of nausea when looking at schoolbooks, the therapist taught English basic grammar using the English instructions for a war game he enjoyed. He learned it even though the process was slow. M was ashamed that he did not know mathematics at the elementary school level. He was then taught fractions and decimals using the same instruction, and he learned them. He occasionally sighed, saying, "The ship has left me behind. Everyone else is far ahead. I cannot bring the past back." He told the therapist, "You're devoting yourself for nothing. I'll be like this forever. How old are you? You will either give up on me or get old and senile."

As if in accord, his mother said to the therapist, "Some people are just scum. If I decided to give him up forever, I could move to a new place and get promoted. Even his parents have gotten sick of him; you are strange." The therapist answered, "Thinking of the future, we do what we can do right now, step by step. It brings the future. I won't give up. I know M is stubborn, but I am the mother of stubbornness." M, unconvinced, said sarcastically, "Sure," but his expression showed some relief with this reassurance.

Studying during therapy sessions was not enough to allow M to catch up, so M requested that a therapist tutor come once a week. This tutor, T, was a gentle male graduate student who was seeking his own identity, changing his major from physics, to medicine, to pharmacology. T listened quietly to M's critical remarks, frankly admitted that he himself hadn't played at all as a child, always studying for entrance examinations. Being good company for M, the therapist tutor truly enjoyed fishing, games, trains, and movies. It surprised M and changed his conception about people. "He is an elite but so lovable. He is a bit strange, but maybe people are not so frightening after all," M said.

M no longer cut off the cat's whiskers, and the cat began to join the family. M kept the fish he caught, as well as finches, as pets. He took such good care of them that the original pair of finches produced a family of 26 birds. Although he occasionally teased or harassed them, by caring for the pets he learned how to relate to animals and people, being friendly but not intrusive. When M decided to go to school though still afraid of group life, he gave each of his acquaintances a pair of finches as a gift to commemorate his starting again.

Entering the Outer World: Recapturing Childhood and Adolescence
(First Semester of Ninth Grade to Entering University)

From the beginning the therapist had contacted the school at the end of each semester. The school had sent M notes and study materials to show that he was welcome to return to class, but the teacher had not urged him to attend school, believing that M was not yet ready. At the beginning of ninth grade, the teacher thought that finally the time was right, visited M's home to invite him to go to school, and promised to meet him at the school gate in the morning.

M's remark about his ninth grade classmates was: "Everyone is OK, but they are so cheerful and have nothing to worry about. I feel left out and cannot join them." He attended school, although he was absent periodically.

Just before M was to graduate, his parents regretted and apologized that they had given up the responsibility for M and left all the responsibility for caring for M to the therapist, which was "therapy by commission." They discussed with M, and decided with him, that M would transfer to the ninth grade of a night junior high school[1] to enjoy real school life, instead of graduating from junior high school by the principal's special approval.

In the night junior high school, M met students with various backgrounds and experiences, and he had a good teacher. He was elected to a class office. M had many experiences, including taking care of a friend who was absent from school, visiting Hiroshima alone and thinking about peace, and playing mischievous tricks with his friends. His parents observed, "He is having a free and natural life as a child. The life we used to have cannot be called a family life. He has seemed to reclaim and enjoy all the childhood pleasure at once." They watched over him leniently.

M became a positive young man capable of leadership and attended part-time high school[2] while working. He proceeded to the science department of a national university. The parents visited the therapist together to report this development and said, "We learned from you not to give up. We hadn't learned it before. We also learned that a husband and wife must find something good in each other and help each other. M suffered for a long time and helped us understand it." While M's father was talking, the mother was nodding at his words with a smile on her face. They looked harmonious.

Discussion and Recommendation for Treatment

School Refusal Children and Their Families

In 19 of the 30 cases we studied the father's participation in the family was minimal (Father < mother in Table 1). This group includes only those cases where it was obvious that the father retreated both physically and psychologically. In the remaining cases, it was difficult to say that the father was considered a good guardian or the

---

[1] The night junior high school was established for adults who did not complete the junior high school course.
[2] The part-time high school was established to meet the needs of students who have diverse life situations.

source of authority in the family. Conversely, in these cases the mother often interfered or gave overzealous care, which was not optimal for the child's mental and physical development or needs. In other words, there was a tendency for the mother not to keep the psychological distance from the child that is appropriate for the child's age. From this perspective, school refusal children are more or less dissatisfied with relationships with their parents, feeling lonely and helpless. Such a situation might cause difficulty in identity development.

Within the family, these clients appear to be the most fragile and defenseless psychologically (and sometimes physically) of all the family members. The client seems to represent the problems the family have experienced, which sometimes have lingered in the family for three or four generations. The symptoms of the child could be considered symbols of the family's problematic situation and a cell for help.

In a family that functions too poorly to raise and care for children, the child's development might not be normal and his or her adaptability to reality might not fostered. When there are many problems to cope with, both externally and internally, such a child cannot manage and may become seclusive and withdraw into his house or room. This situation in turn results in school refusal.

Individualized, Multifaceted Approach for School Refusal

First Interview

Ogura [8] pointed out that the first encounter with the client is significant in terms of determining the process and results of therapy. My experience with 30 cases confirms the importance of the first encounter.

The first requirement is for the therapist to maintain a stance on the same level as the client, not being manipulative. In addition, it is necessary for the therapist to be eager to grow with the client, in both human and professional terms. Although the therapist should have information about the client, it is important to understand the client based on the encounter, disregarding any prior information. To solidify the relationship the therapist should determine some "windows of the heart" in order to establish a therapeutic alliance. This area requires a flexible attitude and allows the therapist to see or think about matters from several perspectives. The therapist must communicate with the child not only through language but by sharing activities (sports, studies, and so on). An interest in youths and their current popular culture is desirable. The ability to readily admit contradictions within one's self is also necessary for successful therapy.

Second, appropriate judgment about whether to accept a case is essential. The therapist must consider if reference to a medical or other type of clinic is needed. It must be decided if a particular clinic is appropriate for the client, considering the facilities in that clinic and the therapist's own ability.

Third, the family must be considered. The therapist must appreciate the worries parents have been experiencing because their child has been absent from school and their efforts to correct the problem [9]. Without identifying who caused the trouble or who the victim is, the therapist must listen to what they have to say. The therapist emphasizes what can be done now and in the future and then foster a cooperative attitude to restore the family.

There are several difficulties that parents experience.

1. They are unable to understand the child's behavior and do not know how to cope with it.
2. They have little interest in the child.
3. They are psychologically caught up in the child's problem and cannot make a proper judgment about it.
4. They have their own serious problems, which distort their judgment and relationship with the child.

In the case of items 1 and 2, the therapist can help parents to understand the child. In the case items 3 and 4, it is necessary to resolve the parents' anxiety first. In reality, these difficulties overlap. In any case, concrete information and hope, based on facts from the assessment, are essential for therapy.

Therapeutic Strategy

The essence of the therapy is not just to urge the child to back to school but to help the child recapture hope in order to grow up, clarify the child's ideas about the life he or she is going to lead, and help the child understand the kind of adult he or she can become. For this purpose, a concrete means is needed to ensure the time and space required so the child can grow again. The first step is to find the client's interests, the "windows of the heart," which the therapist can share and relate to, and to determine what can actually be done now.

Instead of pushing the client into an established form of therapy, it is necessary to invent and employ techniques according to his or her condition. The one-to-one relationship between therapist and client is not the only way to help the child. A therapeutic network, including therapist tutors and group activities for participating in life experiences, is also needed.

Periodic contacts with the school, with the child's and family's consent, is beneficial. When talking to the teacher on the phone, the child could be situated next to the therapist. Also it could be helpful for classmates or the teacher to visit the child's home or to accompany the child to school. The effectiveness of these measures depends on when and how they are undertaken. To utilize the resources in school, the therapist must accurately perceive the client and the situation around him or her.

Regarding consultation with the family, we accept the family situation as it is. A change in the child sometimes moves not only the parents but also the grandparents or brothers and sisters to come for consultation, which may alter the family configuration. There are also cases (as shown in Table 1) where the consultation with the mother or the father alone brings about changes in the family and the child. It is important to respect and foster the client's and the family's autonomy in order to restore their lives.

Termination

In principle, the decision to terminate therapy is the client's responsibility. In some cases, even though the child returns to school, he or she still suffers from many problems. In other cases, having agreed to go back to school, the client goes through significant personality development and is able to determine how to lead his or her own life. A therapeutic goal is for the client to believe that, "I faced a big task and managed to cope with it. In the years ahead I must face many problems, but I will deal with them as necessary."

Concluding Remarks

The treatment for school refusal has several overlapping components: first, providing clients with a snug "nest" in which they can heal themselves and grow again psychologically; second, providing the opportunity to make up for the lack of social learning experiences; and third, making contact with and obtaining the cooperation of the school in order to prepare the child to return to that school. It is essential to offer the family a chance to recognize the natural ties between parents and child and to give the child an opportunity to be psychologically independent from the parents.

Acknowledgments. I appreciate the help and cooperation of my colleagues, co-therapists, and students in the life experience group at Taisho University Counseling Institute. In particular, I would like to thank Assistant Professor Ken-ichi Ito and therapists Kyoko Kato, Humiko Kurihara, and Takako Oyama.

References

1. Iida M, Kasahara Y, Kawai H, Saji M, Nakai H (eds) (1983) Mental science 7: the life cycle (in Japanese). Seishin no kagaku 7, raifusaikuru. Iwanami, Tokyo
2. Murase K, Ito K (1986) Japanese family pathology (in Japanese). In: Shimazono Y, Hozaki H (eds) Seishinka mukku 14, seishonen no shakaibyori. Kanehara, Tokyo, pp 14–25
3. Iida M, Kasahara Y, Kawai H, Saji M, Nakai H (eds) (1983) Mental science 6: the family (in Japanese). Seishin no kagaku 6, kazoku. Iwanami, Tokyo
4. Murase K (1981) Therapeutic development in child psychotherapy: aims and termination (in Japanese). In: Shirahashi K, Ogura K (eds) Tiryokankei no seiritsu to tenkai. Seiwa, Tokyo, pp 19–52
5. Yamanaka Y (1978) Juvenile seclusion: adolescence, psychopathology and therapy (in Japanese). In: Nakai H, Yamanaka Y (eds) Shishunki no seishinbyori to tiryo. Iwasaki-gakujutu, Tokyo, pp 17–62
6. Murase K (1979) The function of a therapist tutor in child psychotherapy (in Japanese). Taisho Daigaku kaunseringu kenkyujo kiyo 2:18–30
7. Bettelheim B (1963) Love is not enough. Macmillan, New York
8. Ogura K (1983) The first interview (in Japanese). In: Yamanaka Y, Nozawa E (eds) Shokai mensetsu. Seiwa, Tokyo, pp 53–92
9. Bettelheim B (1987) A good enough parent. Knopf, New York

Study on the Experience of Being Bullied: Children Refusing School Who Resort to Violence Within the Family

Shuji Honjo

Summary. The issue of bullying among school-age children has become a focus of public concern in Japan in recent years, and the problem has become a frequent topic of media attention. Accompanying this trend, expectations are rising that members of our profession can intervene in some way. Such bullying is not necessarily a new phenomenon, and it is fact that we have frequently encountered bullying as the triggering point for onset of school refusal and other such problems during the course of every day practice. In this chapter the problem of bullying is reviewed through study of 10 subjects with school refusal who also exhibited intrafamilial violence with whom the author has worked intensively. In six of the ten cases, the experience of being bullied was recognized as the turning point for onset of school refusal. And the experience of being subjected to violence or discrimination during infancy or early childhood—shared by many of these subjects—is regarded as a significant trigger for school refusal in a large proportion of these cases. Such experiences are believed to have stimulated the onset of persecutory internal object images in the children's inner world, making the subjects perceive the outer world as being full of threats. Under such conditions, the experience of being bullied is believed to have been a perfect trigger for reactivating their internal persecutory images, making bullying the most appropriate trigger for bringing about their school refusal.

Key words. School refusal—Family violence—Experience of being bullied

The issue of bullying among school-age children has become a focus of public concern in recent years, and expectations are rising for members of our profession to intervene in some way. During the past few years a number of reports have taken up this problem [1–3]. However, this phenomenon is not a new issue, and in fact we have frequently encountered complaints of bullying as the triggering factor for the onset of such problems as school refusal during the course of our everyday practice.

Inherent to the problem of bullying there are those who bully and those who are subjected to the bullying. For the prevention of bullying, it is important to search widely to identify not only the personal factors but problems such as those regarding family, school, and society in terms of those who bully and then work to remove the

Department of Clinical Studies for Family Development, Nagoya University School of Education, Furo-cho, Chikusa-ku, Nagoya 464, Japan factors that give rise to the bullying. With regard to such problems on the part of those who bully, Nagahata et al. [4] reported on an analysis that considered nine such cases, although it is the rare case in which we become involved with children who do the bullying in our daily practice. The common case in which we encounter the phenomenon is the subject who came to exhibit such problems as school refusal, with the experience of being bullied as the trigger. Hence it appears that an appropriate course of action is to pursue the significance of the experience of being bullied in such cases.

I have long been intrigued by the problems of intrafamilial violence and school refusal and have reported on the characteristics of school refusal subjects who also exhibit family violence [5, 6]. It is not uncommon to find the experience of being bullied as being the triggering factor for the onset of symptoms in such cases. In this chapter the psychopathological significance of the experience of being bullied is clarified by taking up this aspect in ten such cases of school refusal with accompanying family violence with which I have dealt relatively intensively.

Case Studies

Table 1 gives the general characteristics of the 10 subjects included in this study. Among these subjects the experience of being bullied was recognized as being involved in some way as the turning point for symptom onset in six (subjects 1–6).

Subject 1 is a boy who was 14 years old at first presentation and who had had the experience of being bullied: He was pressed for money at knife-point, and humiliated in front of friends through such acts as having his pencil case dropped deliberately. Subject 2 is a boy, 11 years old at his first visit, who had been repeatedly kicked around by gangs. Subject 3 is a girl who was 15 at first presentation and who ceased going to school because boys in school had called her repulsive and avoided her. Subject 4 is a boy who presented at 16 years of age. He had been enrolled at a boarding school for junior high students but had been threatened into handing over money and subjected to beating and kicking. He was finally unable to go to school and transferred to a local junior high school. There too, however, he was teased by peers, who said, "The abandoned child returns!" resulting in full-blown scuffles. Subject 5 is a boy who was 14 at his first visit. He was unable to go to school, tired of always having to be on the lookout for bullying. Subject 6 is a boy who was 13 at first presentation and who cited bullying as the reason for not going to school.

Case 1

This boy was 14 years old at first presentation on 18 August 1981. The chief complaints were school refusal, intrafamilial violence, and loss of appetite.

The family consisted of six members: the parents, an elder sister, the subject, and two younger brothers. The father is a principal member of a certain religious organization. The mother is also involved in missionary work in addition to being a housewife. In terms of personality, the subject is quiet and, though capable of taking notice of the finer aspects of life, also possesses an egoistic and stubborn side, which would, for instance, make him keep nagging and doing mischief until he got what he wanted.

Growth History and History of Current Disorder

The father was busy during the subject's infancy and had almost no contact with the subject. However, if the father were to learn upon getting home late at night that the

Table 1. Summary of cases.

Subject	Age at first presentation (years)	Symptoms	Characteristics of growth history	Bullying experience serving as turning point for onset
1 (O.K.), male	14 (grade 9)	School refusal, family violence, physical symptoms (headaches), obsessive symptoms, psychosomatic tendency	Frequently subjected to physical punishment during infancy	Held at knife-point by classmates demanding money; subjected to humiliation in front of friends, e.g., having his pencil case dropped deliberately
2 (K.F.), male	11 (grade 5)	School refusal, family violence, physical symptoms (headaches, stomachaches)	Little contact with father; father frequently violent in home	Beaten and kicked by gangs
3 (O.K.), female	15 (grade 9)	School refusal, family violence, physical symptoms (headaches, etc.), hyperphagia, obesity	Treated with discrimination by father and grandfather in comparison to elder sister	Being called repulsive and treated with disdain by boys in school
4 (M.M.), male	15 (grade 9)	School refusal, family violence	Adopted, though registered as natural offspring during infancy; called an abandoned child behind his back from early childhood	Subject to beating and kicking and threatened to hand over money; harassed with "the abandoned child returns!"
5 (M.T.), male	14 (grade 9)	School refusal, family violence, thamuria	Constant trouble between the father and his mother's grandparents	Ceases going to school; pained by always having to be on the lookout for bullying; actual content of bullying unknown
6 (T.H.), male	13 (grade 8)	School refusal, family violence	—	Cites experience of being bullied as the reason for not going to school, although specifics are unknown
7 (O.T.), male	12 (grade 6)	School refusal, family violence, physical symptoms (headaches, etc.), obsessive symptoms	Subject to violence such as being strangled by his father during infancy	—
8 (K.K.), male	15 (grade 10)	School refusal, family violence, obsessive tendencies	—	—
9 (K.M.), male	13 (grade 8)	School refusal, family violence (stomachaches, etc.), obsessive symptoms	Incidents in which the subject could not cease crying; being punished or having bath water thrown over him by his father	—
10 (H.Y.), male	14 (grade 9)	School refusal, family violence, psychosomatic symptoms, obsessive symptoms	Father's suicide when the subject was in 7th grade	—

subject had been bullying his little brothers he would drag the subject out of bed and beat or otherwise reprimand him. With a repetition of such incidents, the subject came to harbor fear toward his father. Additionally, during infancy the subject spent most of his time with his mother and sister in the house and was not permitted to play with children in the neighborhood. Not enrolled in kindergarten, he was abruptly placed in first grade, where he was frequently bullied and unable to get along with his peers.

The family moved when the subject was starting fifth grade, incurring a change in schools. The subject would repeatedly do things such as promise to play with three groups of friends at the same time, making him break his promise with two of the groups, which made him an outcast among his peers and the target of unpleasant pranks. Asked about this turn in events, the subject stated that he was unable to turn anyone down when invited by friends.

Once he arrived in junior high school there were no particular problems during his first year, but in his second year he was threatened for money at knife-point by two classmates. He was also humiliated in front of his peers through actions such as having his pencil case dropped deliberately. For this reason he ceased eating breakfast from around 20 November 1980 and began to skip school, complaining of stomach-aches, headaches, and the like. Told by teachers to bring his son to school, the father at times dragged the subject to school, after locating his hiding place. Beginning around January 1981 his tendency of school refusal became more pronounced, accompanied by death wishes; and he was often found wandering along the river and other such places after voicing his wish to die.

For that reason, the subject was brought to a psychiatric clinic at hospital "A," where treatment consisted only in persuading him to go back to school. Because he continued not going to school, he was taken to a psychiatry clinic at hospital "B" on March 5. It was recommended that he be hospitalized, and he was admitted to a university hospital on March 16. On the second day of hospitalization he escaped following his mother's visit, but the incident was dealt with simply as a discharge. From about that time, the subject started acting violently toward his sister and brothers, beating and kicking them. Wanting to buy things incessantly, he would demand items such as bicycles and clothing; when denied, he would break things, turn violent to his brother to the point of injury, or yell. With regard to his having been bullied by friends, he expressed a wish to become strong and so took up boxing with a sandbag and practiced the Chinese martial arts. Around April he once flew out of the house with a knife in hand, saying he was going to kill a friend. In May, although his violence appeared to be on the decline, he started showing concern over gaining weight and began limiting his intake of rice, sugar, fruit, and other such foods. Furthermore, he purchased an outlandish school uniform such as that worn by some male school pep-rally leaders in Japan and began using expanders as a display of strength.

Under such conditions, the subject was taken to hospital "C" on August 17 by his parents, who wanted him hospitalized because of his extreme violence. Advised to consult Nagoya University, he was brought into the Psychiatry Clinic at Nagoya University Hospital on August 18.

Course of Therapy

The therapeutic relationship spans a period of approximately 12 years. After about 8 years spent in seclusion, the subject undertook the challenge of the high school graduate equivalency examinations. Passing them, he then gained entry into a university. Commuting to classes from a boarding house, he is spending his life as a college student without any expressed problems and is believed to have just about completed the transition back into society.

The problematical point that became clear through the years of therapy is the subject's extreme fear toward the outer world. For example, the subject stated the following in an interview on 17 February 1984, two and a half years after the start of therapy:

I believe I woke up around 1 a.m. Then I believe I heard noises like someone crunching a paper bag outside. Then I believe the noise continued for a long time. I believe I figured that it could only be a vagrant or somebody who would be doing such a thing at that time of night. The realization made my heart race, and my body started to shiver, then I believe that someone started to kick the fence surrounding the house. A large rock would be thrown against the bathroom wall, and the bathroom would emit tearing sounds. I believe I thought that the person doing such things must be someone with a grudge, or someone who was mentally deranged. I always say big things like I'm going to let loose a round of shots with a shotgun, but when something happens in reality, it's difficult to do anything. The person would tear apart the roof, and throw rocks at my second-floor window. I remember thinking that the person must already have gotten my father and mother downstairs. Around 4:30, I went downstairs to my father and mother's room, and in reality, it was only the sound of snow falling off the roof. But it was the first time I had ever been that scared. I thought it would be embarrassing if the whole family were slaughtered and we were to appear in the newspaper. I really thought it was the end.

To comments from his therapist that "You seem to be constantly afraid that someone is going to get you," he replied, "I've thought that this is it—I can't take any more—many times, but other people don't feel that way. There are times that I ran home simply for having my pencil case fiddled with at school, feeling that that was it, that I couldn't take any more. Just having a book stolen also makes me think that everything is over, when all I really need to do is simply tell the teacher." On 18 October 1985, more than 4 years into therapy, he commented, "Nowadays, telephone pranks and creaking sounds get me scared, thinking that there may be someone in hiding. There were a few phone pranks before, and ever since, I've been scared every time the phone rings. It doesn't bother me during the daytime, but in late afternoon, I get so scared—the phone ringing brings back memories of being bullied long ago as a child."

As described above, the subject was possessed by extreme anxiety that others in the outer world wished to harm him, making him constantly brace himself toward the outer world. It is clear that this anxiety is closely related to his experience of being bullied, which became the trigger for his school refusal. However, as noted by the subject himself, his experience of being bullied, which was perceived as extreme threats to the subject, could have been passed by without being taken so seriously. The background that made the subject take the experience of being bullied so seriously is believed to have been established within the subject prior to being bullied. In other words, it is inferred that the bullying overlapped with the subject's feelings of being threatened by the outer world, bringing about the looming anxiety within the subject. Viewing the subject's experience of being bullied in this light enables one to appreciate the condition in which the subject had remained "holed up" within the home for about 8 years even though the objective environment had completely changed from that in which the subject was bullied.

Analysis of the background in which the subject came to harbor such obsessive fear toward the outer world from early childhood indicated his family environment during infancy to be of great significance. Specifically, the subject spent most of his time prior to entry into elementary school with his mother and sister, and so his social development was delayed. The subject was therefore at a great disadvantage in terms of dealing with his classmates upon entry into elementary school, which became a source of great pressure. In addition to this situation was the even greater significance of his relationship with his father: Although contact between the subject and his father was limited from early infancy, what little contact there was often took the form of violence. Regarding his experience during the elementary school years, the subject noted that "My mother would always be nagging me. She would keep me up until Father came home. And then I would be hit or thrown around, you see. I would be made to stand, and Father would be seated in a chair glaring up at me. When Father moved his hand even slightly, I would cringe, you see. These things are coming back to me gradually these days." Repetition of such experience from early infancy is believed to have built up the fear harbored by the subject against the outer world. It is believed that when the experience of being bullied was compounded by this background, the experience came to be perceived as a critical threat by the subject, to which he responded by attempting to defend himself by withdrawing from the school environment—school refusal.

Needless to say, for such fear toward the external world to be established within the subject, factors other than his experience of being on the receiving end of violence from his father, such as his earlier relationship with his mother and that between his parents, are of vital importance, although these points are not pursued herein.

Discussion

Subject 1 was discussed in detail in order to explain how the experience of being bullied in school could be perceived as a critical threat by overlapping the experience to which a child was subjected during infancy, such as having been treated with violence by the father.

This situation was noted for many of the subjects in this study. For instance, subject 2 is an only child with fundamentally strong mother–child bonding. In contrast, the father had avoided becoming involved in family matters, but when something unpleasant arose at the office he would lose his temper at home for minor reasons, throwing things around and behaving violently at times. In other words, the father was frequently impulsive and uptight in front of his family.

For subject 3, the grandfather treated the subject's elder sister with great affection while showing an obvious dislike for the subject. The father was also fond of the elder sister and had been actively working to place the sister in a private school at the elementary school level. Such experiences ingrained in the subject the feeling of being disliked and discriminated against, which is believed to have been the basis on which her oversensitive reaction to being treated with aversion by male students in school was founded. This point was also noted in her relationship with the therapist, in which she was adamant that she was being discriminated against by her physician, to such a degree that her complaint was sometimes close to being a delusionary conviction.

Subject 4 is a boy who is listed on the family register as natural offspring but who in reality was adopted as a baby. He experienced being called an abandoned child by a teacher in kindergarten and developed alopecia areata about 6 months after entering kindergarten. This subject had received discriminatory treatment since infancy before he began to exhibit school refusal brought on by being bullied in junior high school.

Subject 5 came from a family who had been living in the mother's parents' household since shortly after the subject was born. The father never got along with the mother's parents, and after endless quarreling the family was thrown out of the house when the subject was in sixth grade. The parents were also at odds, and the mother was constantly nagging and interfering with her son. During interviews the subject noted that "What I recall most from the past is being scolded by my mother. It appears the distortion arises from that experience." He frequently complained of feelings of being overwhelmed by his surroundings and of being chased.

A clear experience of having been the subject of violence or discrimination was not evident for subject 6, but the mother was of unstable character with acute mood swings who disliked going out because of the fear of being disappointed by others. The subject spent the first 4 years of his life closely aligned with his mother, a situation that changed only when his younger brother was born. It is inferred that it was difficult for feelings of reliance on the external world to have been solicited under such conditions.

Such are the factors that prevented the constitution of reliance on the external world during infancy in the six subjects who had been bullied, which seemed to be immediate cause for the onset of symptoms. Incidentally, such experiences during early infancy are often seen among subjects in whom the experience of being bullied was not the trigger. For instance, in case 7 the mother often looked on aghast as the child, as an infant, was strangled or beaten by the father for being even slightly unreasonable. Additionally, when the subject was 4 years old he was left in the care of his father's parents for 40 days during his elder sister's hospitalization. He was apparently treated badly by his grandparents, so much so that he was in a stupor upon returning home, in a daze and not uttering a word. He became unable to go to the bathroom alone, although he had been independent in that respect before being left with his grandparents, and appeared to be in a state of fear. In case 9, the father was short-tempered and would yell to the point of distraction when angry or would throw around whatever object on which he could lay his hands. The subject spent much time crying endlessly and was subject to actions such as having bath water thrown over him by his father.

Regardless of whether the experience of being bullied in school was the turning point, many cases of school refusal with accompanying family violence have in common the experience of being the subject of violence, discrimination, or other such persecutory experience during early infancy. It is believed that such experiences gave rise to the fear or feelings of being threatened by the external world that were established in such subjects. For these subjects, the experience of being bullied came to be perceived as extreme threats because they overlapped their previous experiences. Withdrawing from the school environment and staying "holed up" in their homes then became their defense against such anxieties. In psychoanalytical terms, such conditions would be the establishment of persecutory internal object images within the subjects owing to experiences such as being the object of violence or discrimination as infants, and the projection of such persecutory images onto the external world, making the subjects perceive the outer world as a place full of threats. Under such conditions, the experience of being bullied led to reactivation of the subjects' persecutory internal object images, making the experience a threat of serious proportions for the subject. As stated before, the fact that these subjects have long held persecutory internal object images accounts for states such as that of case 1 where the subject continued to feel fear toward the outer world, which kept him secluded at home for about 8 years after the start of therapy.

It is believed that in many of the cases of school refusal with accompanying family violence discussed in this study, persecutory internal images were being established from a relatively early period. Being bullied then became the perfect experience for activating such persecutory internal images. In other words, being bullied can be taken as the most appropriate key experience for promoting the onset of symptoms in such subjects. This progression can also be understood to a certain extent because of the simple fact that the experience of being bullied could be determined to be the trigger for the onset of school refusal in six of ten cases (60%) of school refusal with family violence in this study. The triggers in the remaining four cases were an absence from school for more than a week due to illness (case 7), having been unable to go on to the school of his choice (case 8), and not having done his homework (case 9); there was no determinable turning point in case 10. Hence the experience of being bullied was the trigger for onset of school refusal in most of the cases of school refusal in which there was accompanying family violence in this study. The subjects described in this study were those with whom I have dealt relatively intensively; however, that is not to say that these cases are necessarily representative in terms of the triggering factor that leads to the onset of school refusal with accompanying family violence. Nevertheless, in a separate study [6], I discussed triggering events for the onset of school refusal in 23 cases with accompanying family violence. Being bullied was determined to be the trigger in 10 of the 23 cases (43.5%), and there again the experience of being bullied was the most common triggering mechanism for onset of school refusal.

The following is a review of the percentage of general school refusal (school phobia) cases for which the experience of being bullied triggered the onset of the condition. In one of the early studies Tatara [7] stated that "Many cases come to refuse school following temporary absence due to illness or other such reasons, for being forced to eat school lunches, or complain of physical ailments such as headaches and stomachaches in refusing to go to school." Sogame [8] stated that "It is fact that restructuring of classes, transfers to other schools, entering new grades or new levels of schooling, school exam periods and the like often exist as large turning points for school refusal." Practically no mention is made of the experience of being bullied as turning points by these authors. Wakabayashi et al. [9] conducted a survey on the reasons for not wanting to go to school among elementary school children in Nagoya City, although the ages of the subjects are lower than those of the patients reported herein. According to that survey: "intrafamilial problems," "school is uninteresting," and "separation anxiety from the mother" were listed as the primary reasons, with only 3.7% citing "relationship with friends" as being relevant in terms of bullying. Takagi et al. [10] also conducted an analysis on the factors precipitating school refusal. They found that the factors believed to be related to bullying, such as "being criticized by friends," represented 6 of the 80 factors (7.5%) noted. In a more recent study, Komatsu et al. [11] discussed 25 cases of school refusal; the chief complaints were physical in nature, among which 7 subjects (28%) listed being bullied by friends as being the turning point, or trigger, for the onset of their school phobia.

Okazaki et al. [2] conducted an epidemiological survey on school refusal in Shimane Prefecture, in which they pursued the reasons for absence as stated by the subjects themselves (Table 2). The "matters regarding school" category apparently includes problems relating to studying, tests, homework, roles such as class officers, extracurricular activities, lunch, teachers, and the like, with the problem of bullying

Table 2. Reasons cited for absence by children exhibiting school refusal.

Reason	Grades 1–6	Grades 7–9	Grades 10–12	Total
Matters regarding school	4	8	6	18
Relationships with friends	10	14	5	29
Psychosomatic complaints	19	31	10	60
Vague/undefined reasons	9	26	10	45

From [2], with permission.

believed to be included under "relationships with friends." The subjects citing "relationships with friends" as the reason for being absent numbered 29 of 152 (19.1%). Additionally, Takei et al. [12] investigated the problem of bullying in school refusal subjects under 18 years of age who presented at the Nagoya University Psychiatric Clinic between 1982 and 1985. Their study revealed that 45 of 173 subjects (26.0%) with school refusal had experienced being bullied during that interval.

The percentage of subjects with the experience of being bullied as the triggering point for the onset of school refusal are on the rise, according to the studies by Takagi et al. and Wakabayashi et al. around 1965 and the reports by Komatsu et al. and Takei et al. made around 1985. It is believed that this observation endorses the idea that the problem of bullying in the school setting has increased in gravity in recent years, and that bullying is taking on increasing importance as a factor in the onset of school refusal, as pointed out by Wakabayashi et al. [3].

Incidentally, the studies I have undertaken do not differ greatly from those of Komatsu et al. and Takei et al. in terms of year of execution; but there is a tendency in my study for a larger proportion of subjects who had had the experience of being bullied as their trigger for the onset of school refusal to also have displayed violent behavior within the family. Furthermore, according to data compiled by the Nagoya University Psychiatry Clinic, among the 45 subjects with school refusal who had had the experience of being bullied, 13 (28.9%) had also been reported as resorting to intrafamilial violence. In contrast, among 132 school refusal cases without the experience of having been bullied, only 23 (17.4%) also displayed violence in the family. Thus there was a higher tendency for school refusal subjects who had experienced being bullied to also have displayed family violence ($P < 0.10$) [13].

These data appear to indicate that, when comparing school refusal cases in general, for those subjects also exhibiting violent behavior within the family the experience of being bullied is perhaps the most likely factor for triggering their psychopathological problems. In other words, as I have stated previously, a large proportion of school refusal cases with accompanying family violence, compared to their nonviolent counterparts, have in common the experience of being subjected to violence or discrimination during infancy and early childhood with the subsequent establishment of persecutory internal object images. For such subjects, the experience of being bullied readily provokes persecutory anxiety, making this experience the ideal trigger for the onset of school refusal.

From this viewpoint, it is thus vital to interpret the experience of being bullied in such cases in terms of the subjects' growth history, including the parent–child relationships and environmental conditions. Consideration of the experience of being bullied against the backdrop of the subjects' growth history is the key to shedding light on the meaning and significance of the experience for the subject. As stated with regard to case 1, it is only through such analysis that we can fully appreciate the condition wherein such subjects continue to remain secluded in their homes, finding it difficult to return to society and requiring many years in therapy long after they are removed through graduation, transfers, or the like from the direct conditions under which they were bullied.

Summary

Ten cases of school refusal with accompanying family violence were considered in this study. The experience of being bullied was recognized as the triggering point for the onset of school refusal in 6 of the 10 cases. It was also noted that a large proportion of such subjects had in common the experience of being subjected to violence or discrimination during infancy and early childhood. In this situation, the persecutory internal object images established in such subjects were recognized as being a factor of vital importance when determining the way in which the bullying was to be perceived by the subject. Such recognition is crucial for a therapeutic success.

Acknowledgment. The author expresses sincere gratitude to Prof. Shinichiro Wakabayashi, Department of Neuropsychiatry, Gifu University, for his help in reviewing this manuscript.

References

1. Fujiwara T (1986) The sociopathological problems of adolescents in modern-day Japan—with focus on the problem of bullying. In: Psychiatry MOOK, No. 14: Adolescent sociopathology (in Japanese). Kanehara, Tokyo, pp 1–13
2. Okazaki T, Onoda K, Inagaki T, Kodaki N (1980) An epidemiological approach to school refusal in Shimane Prefecture (in Japanese). Jpn J Child Adolesc Psychiatry 21:333–342
3. Wakabayashi S, Honjo S, Sugiyama T, Ohtaka K, Abe T, Aoyama T, Nawa M, Takei Y, Inoko K, Kaneko T (1986) Psychiatric study of "ijime" [bullying or abuse by class-mates] in child and adolescent (in Japanese). Research-aid paper of the Yasuda Life Welfare Foundation 22(2):184–192
4. Nagahata M, Haibara S, Tanaka S, Ikuse K, Ohno M (1986) A clinical study of bully (Ijime) in primary and middle school children (in Japanese). Psychiatr Neuro Paediatr Jpn 26:79–93
5. Honjo S (1983) The characteristics of school refusal accompanied by family violence (in Japanese). Jpn J Child Adolesc Psychiatry 24:337–353
6. Honjo S (1987) A clinical psychopathological study of the young patients who refuse to go to school and do violence to their family members (in Japanese). Psychiatr Neurol Paediatr Jpn 27:147–176
7. Tatara M (1963) Some observations on school phobia. I. Consideration of the symptom formation (in Japanese). Jpn J Child Adolesc Psychiatry 4:221–235
8. Sogame S (1965) Studies of school phobia. II. Mechanism of symptom formation and residential treatment (in Japanese). Jpn J Child Adolesc Psychiatry 6:157–165
9. Wakabayashi S, Ito H, Ito S (1965) The investigation on the actual condition of school phobia or refusal to attend school (in Japanese). Jpn J Child Adolesc Psychiatry 6:77–89
10. Takagi R, Kawabata T, Fujisawa A, Kato N (1965) Nuclear type of school phobia. I. Symptom formation (in Japanese). Jpn J Child Adolesc Psychiatry 6:146–156
11. Komatsu Y, Tokushige Y, Okuyama M, Toyonaga Y, Hirooka J, Hoashi E, Kumagai K (1982) Children refusing school with physical symptoms as chief complaints (in Japanese). Psychiatr Neuro Paediatr Jpn 22:177–182

12. Takei Y, Inoko K, Wakabayashi S, Honjo S, Nawa M, Kaneko T, Sugiyama T, Ohtaka K, Aoyama T, Abe T (1987) Bullying in terms of school refusal (in Japanese). Jpn J Child Adolesc Psychiatry 28:55–56
13. Wakabayashi S (ed) (1989) Child and adolescent psychiatry—pathology and practice in modern-day society (in Japanese). Kongo, Tokyo

Education and Its Relation to Child and Adolescent Psychiatry: Problem of School Hating

Akihide Kitamura

Summary. In recent years the mental health of Japanese school students, especially at the level of middle school, has become a focus of attention. Teachers are expected to have the skills necessary to attend to the mental health of their students. Herein I discuss the phenomenon of school hating, which is becoming a serious problem in Japan: What is school hating? What are the problems within the educational system in Japan? What are the possible measures for prevention and treatment? Problems of the Japanese school system today are the (1) universality of education; (2) scholastic gaps in high schools; and (3) mental health problems of students as a social phenomenon. School hating is evaluated here by examining (1) statistics on school hating; and (2) school hating at the junior high school level in a particular city, in a public middle school, and the types of nonattending students. Coping with school hating in schools is a problem, Japan's educational system focuses on selecting students according to their scholastic abilities while ignoring their individual personalities. What can we, as psychiatric professionals, do for these students?

Key words. Child and adolescent psychiatry—Elementary and middle schools—School hating

Schools are not only places for studying but also points of entry into adult society. School life forms a world of its own for students.

In recent years, the mental health of Japanese school students, especially at the level of middle school, has become a focus of attention. Teachers are being asked to provide proper and careful guidance to the students at the same time their schedules are becoming busier with the many and various demands of the curriculum. Moreover, teachers are expected to have the skills with which to attend to the mental health of their students. The teacher's role is heavy and demanding.

Under the present school system, there seem to be many maladjusted students, and they and their caretakers are at a loss as to how to correct the situation. They seek help at educational counseling centers for children, visit the mental health departments at health centers, or visit psychiatrists associated with hospitals.

Department of School Mental Health, Nara University of Education, Takabatake-chou, Nara City 630, Japan

The Ministry of Education in Japan defined long-term absentees as those who are absent from school more than 50 days. Among long-term absentees in elementary and middle school, there are long-term absentees who have "cut" their classes for reasons of health or family problems, and there are school haters. Among the school haters are truants (who cut school days because of their delinquency) and nonattendants (who cut school because of school phobia, school refusal, or school dropout).

The phenomenon of "school hating" has becoming a serious problem in Japan. What is school hating? What are the problems within the educational system in Japan? What are the possible measures for its prevention and treatment?

Problems of the Japanese School System Today

Universality of Education

Japan's compulsory education system was based no the Educational System of 1872, the Education Act of 1879, and the School Education Act of 1886. Thus the system has a history of more than 100 years. During these years, the national government had a firm policy of enforcing compulsory education, so that school attendance had reached almost 100% by the end of the Meiji era (1912) (Fig. 1) [1–3]. According to Fujita [4], until the 1920s only the elite received a liberal education. As a result of economic development after World War I, however, more people wanted to go to schools, and the education of the masses became possible. With the high economic growth rate of Japan, education became "universal" in 1955.

After World War II, attendance at middle school became compulsory, and the number of students entering high schools increased rapidly. Today more than 90% of middle students go on to high schools, and more than 30% go on to junior colleges and universities. This is the age of popularized higher education.

Since the 1970s, however, there has been no increase in this 30% rate. The main reason seems to be the economic difficulties of paying for education. Most middle

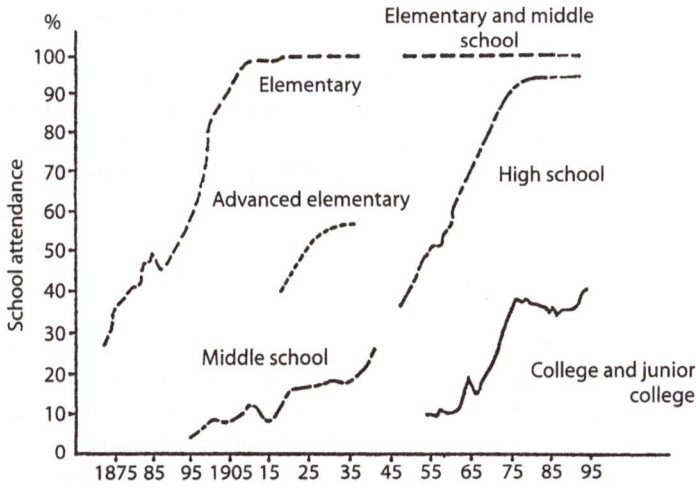

Fig. 1. Changes in school attendance (1873–1993) for elementary school, middle school, high school, and college and junior college

school students go on to enter high schools, a fact that gives the impression that high school education is compulsory. However, there are large gaps in the scholastic levels of these schools, which creates mental health problems for some students.

Scholastic Gaps in High Schools

Because high school education has become semicompulsory and because middle school students go on to high school according to their scholastic abilities, high schools have come to be ranked by their scholastic levels [5], creating gaps. These gaps are so great as to determine not only the child's social status later in life but also his or her view on life. Indeed, the status of the high school attended by students plays a vital role in their life, and yet this status is determined by only two factors: the economic capacity of their caretakers and the scholastic ability of the students. This important educational matter reflects the excessive competitiveness of a society that enforces the choice of school in terms of the economic power of the caretakers and the scholastic ability of students: Neither the student's individuality or humanity nor his or her free will is represented.

At the level of the top high schools, the students are isolated in their competitive struggle for entrance into the better universities. Many of the students become alienated, keeping their personal problems to themselves. In many cases teachers are eager to teach and give guidance about college entrance, but they are unaware of the problems of their students and are certainly not used to paying attention to their mental health. Even those students who do not have problems but who study hard to win the competition may turn out to be unsuccessful in their relationships with others.

On the other hand, at the lower-status high schools, students may suffer when they have difficulty keeping up in class. They may find it difficult to become interested in school life when the only focus is on the curriculum. Thus it is easy for them to acquire antischool behaviors that teachers try to control by force, such as corporal punishment, confinement at home, removal or suspension from school, or poor reports to prospective colleges. The fact that there are 101 000 to 124 000 high school dropouts each year gives some idea of the growing indifference of students and the increasingly strict controls over them.

The problem of status differences, or gaps, among high schools is affecting junior and primary school children as well in the form of harsh competition to attain entry into famous high schools as well as into private, elite middle schools. The popularization of education is now forcing excessive competitiveness and biased scholasticism on children and their caretakers.

Mental Health Problems of Students as a Social Phenomenon

According to Hamada [6], the priority of the Japanese educational system has been to "educate the populace to become able citizens of the State." The concept of the "right" of people to be educated does not seem to have existed. As a result, Japanese education today seems to focus on adherence to group rules, the management of students, and an excessive competition for high scholastic levels; and these characteristics seem to have become even more acute as Japan strides ahead as an economically advanced country.

Needless to say, industrial and economic development demand the high level of knowledge and technology that come from a higher education, and the educational system has worked effectively in providing the necessary education to a large number of people. However, as a result of the overemphasis in all schools on group rules, excessive competition, and a bias toward purely scholastic abilities, education has come to ignore the individuality and humanity of students, which has resulted in the creation of an amazingly large number of students who do not fall into the rigid framework of the school system today. They comprise those students who, because of their personalities, have difficulty submitting to the pressure of group rules and those who are frightened by the excessive competition.

Such problems as delinquency, abuse of organic solvents by inhalation, and school violence arise among middle school students who are not intellectually blessed, or whose families cannot help with their scholastic work. Many of the absentees stop going to school because of fear, and more students are finding the curricula too elaborate and difficult to follow. Unless their families are fully supportive, such children are apt to become maladjusted at school.

A good family atmosphere and careful attention of caretakers to their children's mental health are essential in preventing the development of deviant behaviors. Another requirement is financial support for getting into colleges. Those fortunate children who receive these benefits will gain higher education, and it is they who will fill the positions that influence the national economic and political structures of the future. In the last analysis, although education in Japan is equal for all in principle, in practice it is not based on egalitarianism or true scholarship. The system provides education only to those who are rich, and many children cannot take advantage of the system because of the economically lower status of their caretakers.

The financial ability of the caretaker is the greatest factor influencing the choice of and adjustment to schools, and this situation is causing a polarization into two social strata. At one extreme, students move from wealthy families and educational investment to membership in the governing class of the future. At the other extreme are the students from poor families, who become dropouts and join the class of the governed. Students, teachers, and caretakers are swept along by this current, which brings with it mental health problems for students. These problems, rather than being "illnesses," are social phenomena.

Medical treatment is based on a contract between patients and medical professionals: If patients are not satisfied with the services provided, they can break the contract. Compulsory education, in contrast, is legally imposed on the people by the State as a duty: Students and their caretakers cannot abandon or refuse it even if they believe it is questionable. In fact, it is almost impossible to live without accepting a school education. One of the principal reasons for the various problems that arise in schools today is that school education is forced on the youth by the adult society.

What Is School Hating?

Statistics on School Hating

The Ministry of Education began to gather statistics in 1952 about so-called school hating at the elementary and middle school levels. According to their basic research, the number of students who cut more than 50 school days has been increasing rapidly during the past 20 years, especially at middle schools (Fig. 2). In 1993 the number of

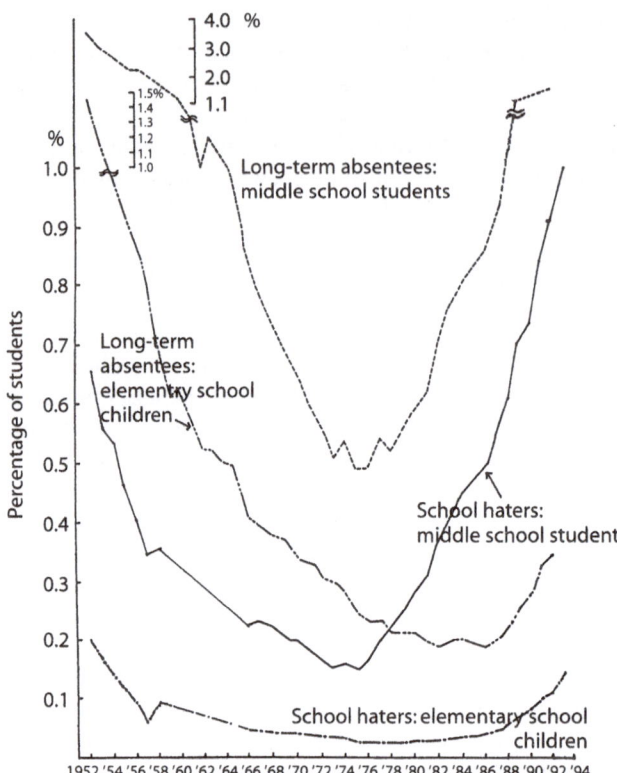

Fig. 2. Long-term absence and "school haters" from statistics by the Ministry of Education (1952–1993). The number of students who are absent more than 50 school days a year has been increasing rapidly during the past twenty years, especially at middle schools

school-hating middle school students reached almost 49 200 (1.01% of the total number of students). Most were cases of truancy and nonattendance.

There are no statistics on school hating among high school students, but it is suspected that the number is even higher. There were about 101 200 dropouts from high schools in 1992 (1.9% of registered students). The major reasons for dropping out of school were maladjustment to school life and studying (26.5%), change in plans for the future (43.3%), and an inability to follow class material (9.9%). Also noticeable is the increase in the number of students who suffer in classrooms because of lack of motivation and those who visit the nurse in the school infirmary complaining of physical symptoms such as headaches and stomachaches.

As shown clearly in Figure 3 [7], the number of school-hating students increases from elementary schools to middle schools to high schools. The subjects of this research were 3 028 227 students (2 039 246 elementary school children and 988 981 middle school children) residing in Osaka, China, Ibaraki, and Shizuoka prefectures. This research was done in 1983, by grades. In these prefectures, 6691 children were cutting school because of school-hating (775 in elementary school, 5916 in middle school). The number increased gradually at the higher grades, and a sudden increase is seen when elementary children began to go to middle school (Fig. 4 [7]), a time when there is a drastic change in the school environment. Because of this major shift in school environment, some children cannot cope with the change and become school haters: Three times more students fall into this category after getting into middle school. A similar phenomenon is seen when middle school students go to high

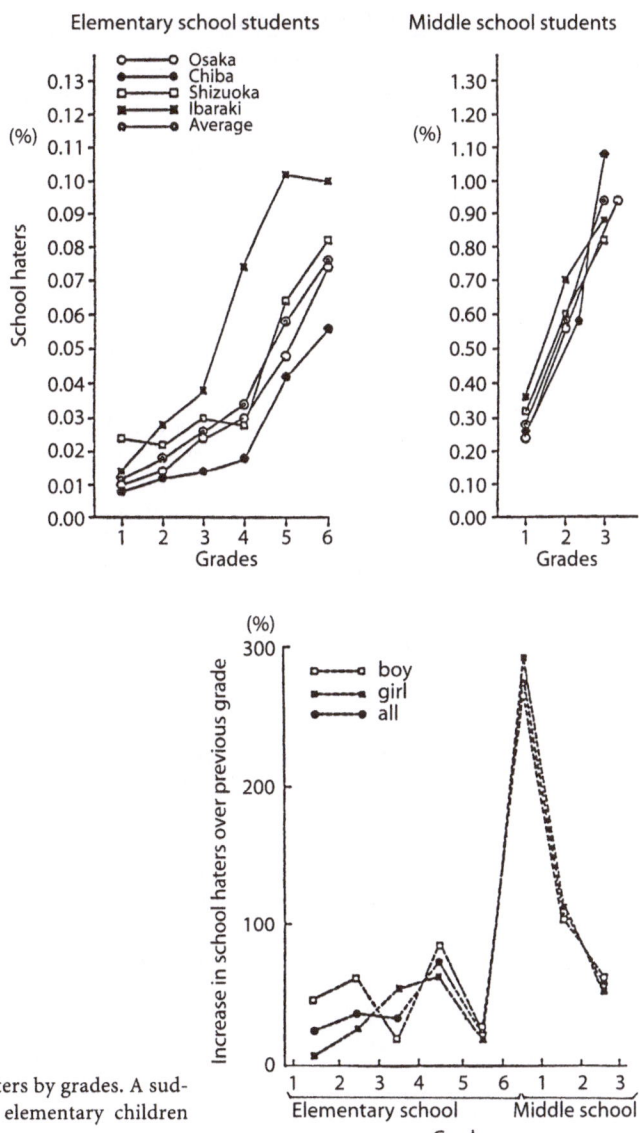

Fig. 3. School haters by grade in four prefectures. The number of school-hating students increase from elementary schools, to middle schools, to high schools, 1983

Fig. 4. Increase in school haters by grades. A sudden increase is seen when elementary children begin middle school

schools, with the largest number of dropouts seen during the first term of the first year. This trend is consistent with the idea that it is a change in the educational environment that is inducing school hating.

School Hating at Middle School

Case of K. City

K. City is a satellite city near a larger one, with a population of about 400 000. According to statistics gathered by the city in 1986 (Table 1), the percentage of school-hating children is high when compared to the national average—about 1.5 to 2.0 times

Table 1. School haters in K. City.

Subjects	Elementary school	Middle school
Boys	9 (0.05%)	92 (0.84%)
Girls	18 (0.11%)	78 (0.78%)
Total	27 (0.07%)	170 (0.81%)

Table 2. School haters in K. City, by grade.

Grade/sex	Rate	Total rate
Elementary school		
Grade 1		
Boys	1 (0.04%)	1 (0.02%)
Girls	—	
Grade 2		
Boys	1 (0.04%)	5 (0.09%)
Girls	4 (0.16%)	
Grade 3		
Boys	1 (0.03%)	2 (0.04%)
Girls	1 (0.04%)	
Grade 4		
Boys	—	2 (0.04%)
Girls	2 (0.07%)	
Grade 5		
Boys	2 (0.06%)	10 (0.13%)
Girls	8 (0.27%)	
Grade 6		
Boys	4 (0.12%)	7 (0.11%)
Girls	3 (0.10%)	
Middle school		
Grade 1		
Boys	13 (0.36%)	27 (0.39%)
Girls	14 (0.42%)	
Grade 2		
Boys	31 (0.87%)	50 (0.79%)
Girls	19 (0.57%)	
Grade 3		
Boys	48 (1.31%)	93 (1.32%)
Girls	45 (1.33%)	

Table 3. Middle school "school haters" in K. City, by section.

Subjects	Section A	Section B
Boys	34 (0.56%)	58 (1.21%)
Girls	25 (0.42%)	53 (1.29%)
Total	79 (0.49%)	111 (1.27%)

higher—for both elementary and middle school levels. In general, higher numbers of school-hating children are found in towns on the outskirts of large cities (i.e., in rapidly changing areas of new housing).

Table 2 shows the trend by grades; note that the numbers increase as the grades go higher: 1.3% of the third-year middle school students are school-haters, which is about 2.7 times more than the national average.

Table 4. Number of absentee students in a middle school.

Category	No. of students	Percent
School refusal		
Boys	27	1.3
Girls	14	0.7
Total	41	1.0
Truancy		
Boys	88	4.2
Girls	35	1.8
Total	123	3.0
Long absence		
Boys	8	0.4
Girls	6	0.3
Total	14	0.3
Totals		
Boys	123	5.9
Girls	55	2.8
Total	178	4.4

Within K. City there are two sections: A, a high-status residential area; and B, where low-income families live (Table 3). In the low-income section B, there are 2.6 times more school-hating students than in the section A. The differences are not only in family background and environment; there are also differences in the content and nature of the school hating itself. I would therefore like to express my view on school hating based on observations of a public middle school.

Case of a Public Middle School

Among the statistics compiled by the Ministry of Education, long-term absentee students are classified in three categories of absenteeism: that due to illness, that due to family problems, and that due to school hating. However, I believe that it is not appropriate to label all the school-hating students as cases of school refusal.

Table 4 shows the number of long-term middle school absentee students whose absence was not caused by illness during the past 20 years [8]. The period of absence is from about 1 week to more than 3 months. The nonattenders and truants in Table 4 are classified as "school refusers and truants." If we define an absence of school refusers and truants as school-hating, the number of school-hating middle school students becomes 4.0% of all students.

Types of Nonattending Students

The reasons for long-term absenteeism are illness or family problems/situation. Another classification for absenteeism is "truancy", and such students are apt to become delinquent. Those students who are not classified as long-term absentees or truants are called nonattending students.

In our clinical experience, we can categorize these nonattending students into three types, as shown in Table 5.

Table 5. Reasons for middle school Absenteeism

Type of absence	Reason for absence
Truancy	Delinquency
Long absence	Illness; Family; Others
Nonattendance	School phobia
	School refusal
	School dropout
	Borderline intelligence

Table 6. Number of students, by symptom.

Symptom	Boys	Girls	Total
School phobia	7	1	8
School refusal	6	6	12
School dropout	7	1	8
Borderline intelligence	7	6	13
Total	27	14	41

Table 7. Characteristics of middle school nonattendance.

Type	Mother–child tie	Assertiveness	Intelligence level	Grades
School phobia	Strong	Strong	Normal or high	Elementary/middle schools
School refusal	Average	Strong	Normal or high	Middle/high schools
School dropout	Average	Weak	Normal	Middle/high schools
Borderline intelligence	Weak or strong	Weak	Low	Elementary/middle/high schools

1. Students who want to go to school but who cannot do so because of anxiety (a phenomenon called school phobia).
2. Students who have their own reasons not to go to school and who continue to refuse to do so . They are not anxious about leaving home but show strong anxiety at school (a phenomenon called school refusal).
3. Students who see no obvious reasons for going to school, see no meaning in school life, and have no interest in school. They stop going to school without realizing when they started to cut school; they are therefore called dropouts, or lethargic nonattenders.

It must be pointed out that when school refusal is discussed the students' scholastic abilities are not touched on. Through our work experience in the field of mental health at middle school and our clinical experience with child and adolescent psychiatric treatment, we have found it essential that we should not ignore the scholastic factor, which influences the phenomenon of nonattendance. Although scholastically borderline students tend to cut school, psychiatric workers do not see them as cases of nonattendance, and so this group is generally ignored. These cases of nonattendance are rarely brought to the attention of counseling centers or psychiatrists.

However, as Table 6 shows, at middle schools there are many such nonattending students who need special guidance. When scholastically borderline students are active and not withdrawn, and when classes are not interesting, many of them become truant and delinquent, and those who are withdrawn and unsociable tend to be nonattenders. They cannot follow the class material and, feeling mentally stressed at school, begin to cut school altogether to become dropouts. If their caretakers, teachers, and therapists force them to go back to school, they obey unwillingly and start to become so tense and anxious at school that they can no longer talk or behave spontaneously, becoming as immobile as robots. Elective mutism is often the result. Table 7 classifies the types of nonattendance in view of separation anxiety, degree of assertiveness, scholastic level, and school grade.

Coping with School Hating in Schools

Table 8 shows what has been done to cope with school-hating elementary and middle school children in K. City. At both elementary and middle school levels, home visits by homeroom teachers and the head of the guidance office are used most frequently as a coping measure. When the visits do not succeed in bringing the students back to school, a considerable number of students are referred to relevant agencies, such as the counseling section of educational centers, child guidance counseling centers (Jidou Soudansho), and youth guidance centers (Table 9). The first two handle most of the cases of nonattendance, and the latter deals with truancy that involves delin-

Table 8. Guidance at school.

Form of guidance	Elementary school		Middle school	
	Boys	Girls	Boys	Girls
During home visits	3	12	80	62
In a special room, not in a classroom			8	5
At a special overnight training session			2	2
Provided by coordinating with other agencies concerned	4	3	21	29
Other				
Student currently attending school		2		1
Checking by telephone	2	2	2	1
Home visit at night			3	
After-school tutoring			3	
Avoiding forcing student		1	1	
Have classmates visit home			3	1
Student refuses intervention			2	2
Verbal guidance			3	
Other			1	2

Table 9. Agencies where guidance is given (actual number).

Agency	Elementary school	Middle school	Total	%
Educational institution	6	19	25	21.2
Guidance counseling center		13	13	11.0
Child guidance clinic center	5	15	20	16.9
Youth guidance center		3	3	2.5
Volunteer members		5	5	4.2
City guidance center		20	20	16.9
Prefectural guidance center		26	26	22.0
Residential institution		6	6	5.1
Total	11	107	118	

quency. Presumably, some of these nonattending students are seeing psychiatrists, but the school statistics do not mention the medical or psychiatric history of the students.

Conclusion

Only the objective facts have been stated here about school hating by children at the elementary and middle school levels, with statistics about their types and coping methods. Japan's educational system focuses on selecting students according to their scholastic abilities, and their individual personalities are ignored; they are strictly managed. Excessive scholastic competition dominates all concerned—teachers, students, caretakers—making them lethargic. Under such circumstances, what can we psychiatric professionals do for such students?

At least, as counselors we should avoid separating them from their schools. We should like to see teachers getting involved in the mental health of their students by acquiring the appropriate skills. Teachers, as professionals in the field of education, have the best opportunity for contributing to their students' mental health. What we can do as psychiatrists is to discuss students' problems with teachers and share our therapeutic knowledge and skills with them.

References

1. National Education Research Institute (1972) A century history of Japanese modern education (in Japanese), vols 3–5. NERI, Tokyo
2. Editorial Committee Gathering Japanese Education Data after World War II (1984) A gathering of Japanese education data after World War II: a separate volume (in Japanese). Sanichi-Shobou, Tokyo
3. Japan Education Ministry (1958, 1966–1993) Statistical report of fundamental investigation of schools (in Japanese). JEM, Tokyo
4. Fujita H (1983) Increase in quantity and change in quality in high school (in Japanese). Gendai no Esupuri 195:25–34
5. Iwaki H, Mimizuka H (1983) General statement about high school students in scholastic gaps (in Japanese). Gendai no Esupuri 195:5–24
6. Hamada Y (1977) Postponement to enter school. In: Yoda A (ed) New encyclopaedia of educational psychology (in Japanese). Kaneko-Shobou, Tokyo, p 375
7. Kitamura A (1986) School education and adolescents—problem in school. Jpn Bull Soc Psychiatry 9:201–207
8. Kitamura E, Kitamura A, Nishiguchi T, Terakawa N, Fukunaga T, Wada K, Nishiura M (1983) Non-attendance of school in a public junior high school over a fifteen-year period. Jpn J Child Adolesc Psychiatry 24:322–336

Nosological Constellation
of School Refusal Syndrome

Masayuki Shimizu

Summary. The nomenclature "school refusal syndrome" is no longer used in the international classification of mental disorders, although it is still used frequently in the psychiatric field of Japan because of clinical convenience. This study was carried out with the idea of clarifying the essential pathological state of so-called school refusal, a disorder of childhood and adolescence. The patients diagnosed as having school refusal syndrome according to Japanese criteria were then characterized using international diagnostic criteria. The study included 34 patients, ranging in age from 10 to 17 years, who had been diagnosed as having school refusal syndrome at the psychiatric ward of our hospital. They were followed for 8 to 15 years, and an attempt was made to determine their lifetime diagnoses according to the criteria of ICD-10. Some misdiagnoses were noted, including schizophrenia in two cases, affective disorder in one case, eating disorder in one case, and mental retardation in one case. Others diagnosed as having the school refusal syndrome in Japan were then classified into three groups: (1) those meeting the diagnostic criteria for adult neurotic disorders (F4); (2) those who had behavioral and emotional disorders with onset usually during childhood or adolescence; and (3) those determined to have personality disorders.

Key words. School refusal—Adolescence—ICD-10—Nosology in psychiatry

The nosological entity school refusal has a history of 60-odd years since when it was first recognized in the field of psychiatric medicine [1, 2]. At present, however, it has been deleted from the international diagnostic classifications known as ICD-10 and *DSM-IV* [3], although the term is still used by Japanese clinical psychiatrists. In Japan various questions arise as to its existence. One is whether school refusal is truly a disease. It would be quite proper that a phenomenon of school non-attendance be considered not a disease but a behavioral pattern of children in a certain cultural circle. Psychiatrists in Japan consider it a disease, reporting school refusal as a clinical entity [4, 5]. The same applies to the phenomenon in England [6, 7]. In Japan, it is recognized as a form of psychopathology with a wide spectrum of manifestations, from a simple aberrant behavior in school to an adjustment disorder or other diseases. I carried out a series of nosological studies related to the school

Mie Prefectural Asunaro Hospital, 1-12-3, Shiroyama Tsu-shi, Mie 514, Japan refusal syndrome in order to determine the psychological factors that led to the disorder.

Subjects and Methods

A total of 34 patients were studied, including 15 boys and 19 girls with ages ranging from 10 to 17 years at the time of their first examination. They were diagnosed as having school refusal during examination at the outpatient clinic of own hospital over an 8-year period.

The follow-up study was conducted by mailing questionnaires to their caregivers. Based on the results of these questionnaires, individual cases were examined again, collecting as much lifetime data as possible. The diagnostic criteria of the ICD-10 for mental and behavioral disorders [3], and, when necessary, the ICD-10 criteria for research [8] were employed.

Results

As shown in Table 1, there were 2 cases of schizophrenia, 1 case of an affective disorders (F3), 10 cases of neurotic disorders (F4), 1 case of an eating disorder (F50), in 4 cases of personality disorder (F6), 1 case of mental retardation (F7), and 13 cases of behavioral and emotional disorders during childhood and adolescence (F9). One case was undiagnosable. Another case with headache, the cause of which was unspecifiable, was transferred to the G-Code as a neurological disorder.

Table 1. ICD-10 diagnoses of 34 patients.

ICD-10 category	Diagnosis	Boys	Girls	Total
F2	Schizophrenia	0	2	2
F3	Affective disorders	1	0	1
F4	Neurotic disorders			
F40.1	Social phobias	1	1	2
F41.0	Panic disorder	0	1	1
F42.0	Obsessive-compulsive disorder	2	0	2
F43.2	Adjustment disorders	1	1	2
F45.0	Somatoform disorders	0	3	3
F5 (F50.0)	Anorexia nervosa	0	1	1
F6	Personality disorders	1	3	4
F7	Mental retardation	0	1	1
F8	Developmental disorders	0	0	0
F9	Behavioral and emotional disorders during childhood and adolescence			
F92.9	Mixed disorder of emotions	1	0	1
F93.0	Separation anxiety disorder	2	2	4
F93.8	Other emotional disorders	3	2	5
F93.9	Unspecified emotional disorders	1	0	1
F94.8	Other social functioning disorders	0	2	2
Others		0	2	2
Total		13	21	34

Schizophrenic Disorders

The patient was a 16-year-old girl at the time of initial examination. She began to stay away from high school when she was 15 years old, taking advantage of an episode of fever and diarrhea. Her parent, who was anxious about school refusal, brought her to the psychiatric department for examination. Treatment was suspended when she started to attend school again. The follow-up study 8 years later revealed that she was admitted for treatment of schizophrenia at age 21; she is now 24 years of age and lives with her father. She has a job in a small workshop run by a relative and has no friends. Upon detailed study of her medical record, it is possible that at the initial examination she might have had early stage schizophrenia; that is, she had had some bizarre episodes, such as suddenly wanting to enter a nunnery, secluding herself in her room without eating, and so on.

She was diagnosed as having hebephrenic schizophrenia (F20.1). If hallucination, delusion, or the first rank symptoms of schizophrenia had been noted at that time, her disease would have been differentiated as schizophrenia or a related disease. Because her isolating-autistic tendency, bizarre behavior, slovenly appearance, and so on are not considered unnatural during adolescence, it may have caused the diagnostician to overlook schizophrenia and its associated disorders, especially when the phenomenon of nonattendance at school is a strong possibility. This case indicates that clinicians should reconsider the diagnosis.

Affective Disorders

The patient was a 15-year-old boy at the time of initial examination. He had been subject to colds since the autumn of the year he was in the third grade of middle school. In high school, too, he had many hypochondriacal complaints and was unable to make friends. Because of his chief complaints of "feeling languid, cannot do the school work and hating to attend school" he was examined by the psychiatrist at age 15, one month after entering high school. Treatment was suspended for a short period. At this point, his problem was diagnosed as school refusal syndrome caused by his inability to adapt to school life and a strong hypochondriacal tendency. After 9 years the follow-up study revealed that he had gone back to school and upon graduation from a national university had became a graduate student, devoting himself to his studies and maintaining good personal relationships.

This patient is assumed to be a case of single mood disorder (F38.0). During the course of his school refusal he was noted to be listless, moody, and tired occasionally. Thus when nonattendance is the focus, the physician might overlook the soft psychiatric sign of an affective disorder, thinking that such asthenic atmosphere is a secondary phenomenon. Another factor that might have caused a misdiagnosis in this case is the fact that the initial examination took place during the 1960s when nearly no one showed an interest in emotional disorders in adolescents. It is necessary to inform clinicians that it is possible for adolescents to have some symptoms of depression even though at a low frequency.

Neurotic Disorders

The category of neurosis is beginning to disappear from the international agenda for clinical assessment in psychiatry. In the present study, however, for the purpose of understanding the spectrum of diseases behind school refusal syndrome the F4 categories of the ICD-10 are expressed collectively as neurotic disorders.

A 12-year-old girl diagnosed as having panic disorder (F41.1) complained at her initial examination that, "I do not like to attend the school feeling unwell," and refused to go to school because she was unable to have breakfast. After treatment for about a year with psychotherapy she was able to attend school again. She finished middle school but then stayed at home, having no job. She was 24 years old at the time of the follow-up study, which revealed that although she lives an ordinary life at home she cannot maintain general personal relationships owing to strong anxiety and not being able to work. Her problem is considered to be a generalized anxiety disorder (F41.1) due to a panic disorder becoming chronic.

There were two cases of obsessive-compulsive disorder among the subjects in this study. Many researchers have noted that there is a trend for anancastic personality traits to be associated with the school refusal syndrome. It is easily understandable that school refusal can be rediagnosed later as obsessive-compulsive disorder. It would depend on whether anancastic personality, obsessive ideas, or obsessive acts, as well as nonattendance, are evident. Thus for the lifetime diagnosis such cases are to be labeled obsessive-compulsive disorder.

There is a category of reaction to severe stress and adjustment disorders, F43, in the ICD-10 system. There is no getting around the impression that it was once categorized as neurosis (especially of unspecified type), which is no longer used today. When a psychopathological behavior with unclear boundaries, such as school refusal, is studied, care must be taken not place it in a "wastebasket" diagnostic category. Even with this cautionary note, two cases fell into this category. There were three cases categorized as somatization disorders. Numerous discussions are available related to the various physical symptoms complained of by the patients with school refusal syndrome [9]. The labels for such cases may change depending on whether the subject has hypochondriacal psychopathology or an adjustment disorder.

Behavioral Syndromes Associated with Physiological Disturbances and Physical Factors

There was only one case belonging to the F5 category (behavioral syndrome with physiological disturbances and physical factors). This girl had anorexia nervosa (F50.0). At the time of the initial examination she already had a desire to be thinner and so was dieting. As it was not a serious problem at that time treatment was given for a trend toward hypotension, low spirit, and school nonattendance as the major problems. From the results of the follow-up study, her disorder was diagnosed retrospectively as anorexia nervosa.

Personality Disorders

Four subjects were diagnosed as having personality disorders (F6). None of the four could be categorized properly by a symptomatic diagnosis, and so they were assigned an F6 diagnosis. When examined at the psychiatric clinic, school nonattendance was the presenting issue, although basically the diagnosis was one of social maladjustment, and the nonattendance at school was considered secondary to the maladjustment. These cases were presumed be similar to that described by Coolidge et al. [10], who called it a character disturbance.

Mental Retardation

A girl, in the second grade of middle school (IQ 74), was diagnosed in the category of mental retardation (F7). Because her IQ was borderline, she could not keep up with the class work or make friends at school, which induced her to stay away from school. After being transferred to a special class for the handicapped, she was satisfied with school life and started to attend again. After finishing middle school she obtained a job and lived a stable life in her own way.

At the level of mild or borderline mental retardation, being poor in intelligence and emotional abilities, some pupils are unable to adapt to school life, which might seem like school refusal at first. In these cases it is necessary to place priority on the educational aspect, rather than offer medical help.

Behavioral and Emotional Disorders with Onset Usually During Childhood and Adolescence

Thirteen cases were considered behavioral or emotional disorders with onset during childhood or adolescence. Among them were 10 subjects who had an emotional disorder with onset specific to childhood. Four of these subjects had a separation anxiety disorder. Hence it is known that there are cases corresponding to the school phobia described by Johnson [2]. Five cases were categorized only as "other" childhood emotional disorder, in which the specific school refusal syndrome in Japan may be involved.

Discussion

It has long been discussed whether so-called school refusal is a disease (a particular clinical entity) or a simple syndrome [4]. Psychiatric debate related to school refusal syndrome is closed in the United states, although it remains open mainly in England and Japan [4–7]. Recent discussions in Japan have begun to recognize that school refusal is rarely considered a nosological entity and, different from other countries, it is considered necessary to leave this clinical entity as a syndrome. It is considered to be a problem derived from the educational administration or social state rather than a psychiatric problem [5].

To understand the psychopathology that manifests as school refusal, it is necessary to grasp the pathological entities or diseases behind the disorder. Several studies are available for this purpose. I have tried to evaluate these diseases indirectly by following up the cases diagnosed as school refusal at the initial examination in terms of the subjects' long-term prognosis.

Two issues arose as a result of the study. One is the number of cases believed to have been misdiagnosed at the initial examination. Those labeled as schizophrenia, affective disorder, anorexia nervosa, or another lifetime diagnosis may have been misdiagnosed. Those related to the earliest stages of schizophrenia or mild depression are occasionally difficult to differentiate from other disorders.

Another issue is the psychopathology behind school refusal. Subjects were roughly divided into two ICD-10 groups: F4 (neurotic disorders) and F9 (emotional and behavioral disorders). These two categories are similar in pathological structure, being differentiated from each other only by the difference in the ages of the patients.

The former diagnosis is assigned to adults or near-adults, whereas the latter is assigned to children and adolescents.

Based on the above results, it is assumed that there are three groups who exhibit the so-called school refusal syndrome: those with anxiety disorders, those with adjustment disorders, and those with personality disorders. There is also a miscellaneous group involving those at some risk of misdiagnosis because they are at an early stage of depression or have various other diseases. I hope to follow up on the background of the school refusal syndrome and so be able to cope with the individual clinical case using the results of this study: psychopathological analyses related to the school refusal syndrome in terms of the lifetime diagnosis.

References

1. Broadwin IT (1932) A contribution to the study of truancy. Am J Orthopsychiatry 2:253–259
2. Johnson AM (1941) School phobia. Am J Orthopsychiatry 11:702–708
3. World Health Organization (1992) The ICD-10 classification of mental and behavioral disorders. WHO, Geneva
4. Shimizu M, Hirayama H (1986) School phobia—is it a disease? Nagoya Med J 31:27–33
5. Shimizu M (1989) The relationship between school refusal and school education. Jpn J Child Adolesc Psychiatry 30:232–238
6. Galloway D (1985) School and persistent absentees. Pergamon Press, Oxford
7. Hersov L, Berg I (eds) (1980) Out of school. Wiley, Chichester
8. World Health Organization (1983) The ICD-10. diagnostic criteria for research. WHO, Geneva
9. Shimizu M, Suzuki Y (1985) Psychosomatic disease in adolescence—from the theme of severeness of school-attendance (in Japanese with English abstract). Shinshin Igaku 25:73–79
10. Coolidge JC, Willer ML, Tessman E, Waldfogel S (1960) School phobia in adolescence: a manifestation of severe character disturbance. Am J Orthopsychiatry 30:599–607

Part 4

Neurotic Disorders

Clinical Study of Conversion Disorders in Adolescents

Shozo Aoki

Summary. Eighteen adolescent patients (14 girls, 4 boys) with conversion disorders were studied. They were divided into three groups according to their personality characteristics, premorbid adaptation, and self-image. Group one (identified as the "active type") were extroverted, active, and competitive, and they showed excellent adaptation. They were leaders, and their positions among their peers were central. Group two (identified as the "passive type") were introverted, passive, and noncompetitive; they showed average adaptation. They were listeners and followers, and their positions among their peers were at the outer periphery. Group three had mixed characteristics. As precipitating factors, peer problems and lowered school marks were explored; and as environmental factors for improvement, experiences of joining noncompetitive groups and acquiring friends of the opposite sex were explored. Thirteen of the patients no longer had conversion symptoms at the follow-up (average 5 years), and 15 of them showed good social adaptation. It appeared that a useful outcome of the treatment was a change in the patient's self-image and self-esteem among the active type patients, whereas these areas needed to be maintained and supported in the passive type subjects.

Key words. Adolescence—Conversion disorders—Dissociative disorders—Follow-up study

In Western countries conversion disorders began to decrease after World War II, and by the 1960s they were uncommon [1]. Studies of conversion disorders during childhood and adolescence suggest that the incidence is rare in the psychiatric field [2–4] but relatively high in the pediatric and pediatric emergency field [5] and in immigrant groups, e.g. from Mediterranean countries [6]. In a more recent study, however, Steinberg found that in an adolescent psychiatric inpatient unit population, somatic symptoms, actual physical disorders, and conversion symptoms are common [7].

In Japan some reports also pointed out a decreasing incidence of conversion disorders [8–10]. Nevertheless, in Japan conversion disorders are still not rare and are seen especially by psychiatrists working in general hospitals among patients referred by general practitioners and specialists.

Department of Neuropsychiatry, Okayama University Medical School, Shikata-cho 2-5-1, Okayama 700, Japan

Based on my own clinical experience, there seem to be two personality types represented among those with conversion disorders in Japan. One group of patients are active and extroverted and are leaders in their peer groups. The other patients are passive and introverted and tend to be followers and listeners in their peer groups. In this study the difference between these two groups in terms of treatment and follow-up was examined, and the opportunity was taken to explore differences between Japanese and Western adolescents in terms of conversion disorders.

Subjects and Methods

Eighteen adolescents (4 boys, 14 girls) with conversion disorders who met the diagnostic criteria of the *Diagnostic and Statistical Manual, Third Edition, Revised (DSM-III-R)* were studied. All were inpatients or outpatients in the Department of Neuropsychiatry at Okayama University Hospital from 1978 to 1985. They were investigated for age, sex differences, family backgrounds, personality characteristics, premorbid adaptation, regard by others, precipitating factors, clinical symptoms, treatment, and environmental factors related to improvement mainly from medical records. Follow-up assessment was done by interview with patients and parents, either in person or by telephone. There was a minimum follow-up interval of 2 years. In all cases, I was actively involved in management and treatment.

Results

Age and Sex Distribution

There were 4 boys and 14 girls ranging in age at onset from 10 to 18 years (mean 14.8 years) (Table 1). Age at first referral was 13 to 20 years (mean 16.3 years).

Table 1. Features of 18 patients with conversion disorders.

Pt no.	Sex	Age at onset (years)	Age at referral (years/months)	Duration of treatment (years/months)	Presence of symptoms at follow-up	Adaptation at follow-up
1	F	13	19/8	0/7	−	Good
2	F	10	15/3	0/1	+	Good
3	F	14	14/7	2/1	−	Poor
4	F	13	13/7	0/1	+	Good
5	F	15	15/10	5/0	+	Poor
6	M	18	18/9	5/5	−	Good
7	M	16	17/0	1/2	−	Good
8	M	14	14/7	0/1	−	Good
9	F	16	18/10	2/0	−	Good
10	F	15	16/0	2/1	−	Good
11	F	14	15/2	4/7	−	Good
12	M	13	13/7	1/6	−	Good
13	F	18	18/3	2/8	−	Good
14	F	17	17/0	2/3	−	Good
15	F	10	15/4	2/5	+	Poor
16	F	15	17/6	0/11	−	Good
17	F	19	20/7	3/8	+	Good
18	F	17	17/8	1/5	−	Good

Family Background

Family history revealed that two of the fathers were alcoholics. One father had a phobic disorder. One mother had an anxiety disorder. As for parental attitudes toward patients, three fathers were violent and three were distant. Nine mothers were overprotective, and seven mothers were neglectful. Four patients had obvious conflicts with their siblings.

Personality Characteristics

Eight patients were cheerful, extroverted, active, and independent (patients 1–8). They were strong enough to compete with their peers. Five of the eight patients (nos. 2, 4, 5, 6, 8) were self-centered and selfish. Six patients (nos. 13–18) were shy, introverted, passive, and dependent. They had a tendency to avoid competing with their peers. Four patients (nos. 9–12) had mixed characteristics of above the two personalities. Most patients liked taking care of small children and small animals. Five of them wanted to be nurses.

Premorbid Adaptation and Regard by Others

Eight patients (nos. 1–8) were the leaders of their classes and clubs. School attainment was high for five of the eight and average in the other three. Their parents regarded them as "good" children who were strong and independent. Their peers regarded them as reliable persons. They were socially well integrated into the peer group. Their positions among their peers were central. In accordance with their personality characteristics, this group was called the "active type."

Six patients (nos. 13–18) were regarded as listeners and followers. School attainment was average in all six. Their parents regarded them as obedient and compliant, and they were thought of as quiet and obedient persons by their peers. Their positions among their peers were at the outer periphery. Again, in accordance with their personality characteristics, they were called the "passive type" group.

Four patients (nos. 9–12) were isolated ("lone wolves"), but their school attainment was high. They had mixed characteristics of the other two groups.

Precipitating Factors

Eight of the patients had problems with peer relationships, such as isolation within the peer group. Five of the patients had problems with low school marks. Three experienced failure in a club activity or a job. One patient experienced his father having a surgical operation. One had a broken love affair, and another had an economic problem.

Clinical Symptoms

Conversion Symptoms

Motor disturbances

Eight patients had gait disturbance (four with astasia-abasia, one with muscle weakness of all limbs, one with right hemiparesis, one with paraplegia of the lower limbs,

Table 2. Clinical symptoms.

Pt. no.	Main clinical symptoms
1	Hyperventilation, headache, self-mutilation (wrist cutting)
2	Paresthesia, visual disturbance (tunnel vision), loss of consciousness, headache, fever, urticaria
3	Abdominal pain, headache, orthostatic dysregulation
4	Syncope, atonia attack
5	Twilight state, loss of consciousness, psychogenic amnesia, eating disorder, blindness, self-mutilation (wrist cutting)
6	Gait disturbance, muscle weakness, paresthesia, visual disturbance (tunnel vision), loss of consciousness, vomiting, dizziness, headache
7	Muscle weakness and paresthesia of all limbs, hyperventilation, eye pain, back pain, low grade fever
8	Convulsion, opisthotonus, loss of consciousness
9	Aphonia, hyperventilation, twilight state, psychogenic amnesia, self-mutilation (wrist cutting, overdose)
10	Muscle weakness and paresthesia of fingers, hyperventilation, orthostatic dysregulation
11	Astasia-abasia, hyperventilation, hiccups, pollakiuria, twilight state, psychogenic fugue, psychogenic amnesia
12	Gait disturbance, muscle weakness and paresthesia of left upper limb, vomiting, hearing disturbance
13	Astasia-abasia, hyperventilation, headache, tinnitus, orthostatic dysregulation, dizziness
14	Twilight state, loss of consciousness, self-mutilation (wrist cutting), auditory hallucination
15	Tremor, writer's palsy
16	Astasia-abasia, hyperventilation
17	Astasia-abasia, hyperventilation, twilight state, psychogenic fugue
18	Paresthesia, muscle weakness, self-mutilation (wrist cutting), auditory hallucination

one with falling); one had muscle weakness of the left upper limb; one had aphonia; and one had a tremor (Table 2).

Sensory disturbances

Five patients had paresthesia of one or more limbs (two of the left upper limbs, one of the right limbs, one of the upper limbs, one of both upper and lower limbs). Four had visual disturbances (two with tunnel vision and two with decreased vision). One had hearing disturbance.

Epileptiform Disturbances

Eight patients had seizures (one with convulsion and opisthotonus, one with atony, and six with loss of consciousness).

Autonomic Nerve Disturbances

Eight patients had hyperventilation syndrome, three had orthostatic dysregulation, two had fever, one had vomiting, and one had urticaria.

Associated Symptoms

Dissociative Symptoms

Five patients experienced the twilight state, and two of five patients had psychogenic fugue

Behavioral Problems

Five patients experienced self-mutilation, and one had an eating disorder.

Psychogenic pain disorders

There were six patients in this category: five with headache, one with abdominal pain, one with eye pain, one with back pain, and one with throat pain.

Treatment

Of the 18 patients, 14 underwent inpatient treatment and four were treated as out-patients. The duration of admission ranged from 2 weeks to 8 months (mean 10 weeks).

For individual psychotherapy, the therapist first tried to support the patients by listening to their efforts carefully and with empathy. In most cases the therapist then tried to guide the patients to some insights about their personality and attitudes toward others and to change them gradually. In most cases a behavioral approach and environmental manipulation were used concurrently.

As medication, levomepromazine was effective in eight patients (four patients were given 20 mg daily, one was given 50 mg daily, two were given 150 mg daily, and one took 600 mg daily). Thioridazine was effective in one patient at a dose of 50 mg daily. Antianxiety drugs and antidepressants were not effective.

Follow-up

The average age at follow-up assessment was 21 years 11 months (June 1987). Follow-up periods after the first referral ranged from 2 years 1 month to 9 years 4 months (mean 5 years 4 months).

Conversion symptoms of five patients (27.8%) disappeared within 1 year and in five others (27.8%) between 1 and 2 years. In eight patients (44.4%) the conversion symptoms continued for more than 2 years. In three patients they disappeared between 2 and 5 years (Table 3). At the time of follow-up five patients (nos. 2, 4, 5, 15, 17) still had

Table 3. Follow-up after first referral.

Resolution of symptoms	No. of pts.	%
Disappeared in 1 year	5	27.8
Disappeared at 1–2 years	5	27.8
Continued for >2 years	8	44.4

conversion symptoms. Two (nos. 2, 17) of the five were diagnosed as having somatization disorders (*DSM-III-R*); the other two (nos. 4, 15) had repeated worsening and recovering. One of these five patients recovered gradually and had slight conversion symptoms at the time of follow-up (Table 1).

In terms of social adaptation, seven patients left school (nos. 1, 2, 5, 9, 15, 17, 18), two others withdrew for long periods (nos. 3, 12), and three stayed in the same grade (nos. 6, 10, 11). At the time of follow-up 15 patients had adapted well and only 3 patients had adapted poorly (nos. 3, 5, 15) (Table 1).

Environmental Factors Related to Improvement

Joining new groups had a good influence on 10 patients (nos. 6–9, 11–14, 16, 18). Five of the ten patients improved by joining small and less competitive groups and attaining good positions in the group (nos. 7, 9, 13, 14, 18). Patient 7 failed to get a good position on the high school baseball team and then joined a less competitive baseball team and obtained a star position. Patient 13 entered a small business school and became a scholarship student. Patient 14 entered a school of domestic science and became an excellent student. Patients 9 and 18 took high school correspondence courses. The common characteristics of these schools and teams were that they were smaller and less competitive.

Five of the ten patients improved after entering a high school or a university (nos. 6, 8, 11, 12, 16) and making new friends and establishing new relationships. These schools were not small but were less competitive.

Patient 10 improved after being elected representative for the student union. Patient 1 improved after leaving a nursing school and going back to her hometown. Five patients improved by acquiring a special friend of the opposite sex (nos. 2, 9, 11, 17, 18). Two of these five patients married these partners.

Case studies

The conversion disorders were typed by the differences in personality characteristics, social adaptation, regard of others, self-image, and self-esteem (Table 4). There were two groups: those composed of the "active type" individuals (patients 1–8) and those comprising the "passive type" (patients 13–18).

Active Type Conversion Disorder (Patients 1–8)

Patient 7

An example of the active type conversion disorder was seen in patient 7, a 17-year-old boy.

There was nothing specific in his medical history, and his personality was cheerful, obliging, and responsible. He had many friends. He was a leader in his peer group, especially in sports.

Family Background

His father was enthusiastic about his son's education. The mother was modest and quiet. He had a younger brother age 15 and a younger sister age 10.

Table 4. Two types of conversion disorder during adolescence.

Parameter	Active type	Passive type
Regard by parents	Good child who is easy to raise; independent of parents	Good child who is easy to raise; obedients; compliant
Position among peers	Central; leader	Outer periphery; listener and follower
Self-image, self-esteem	Good child who is supperior to others; stable self-image; high self-esteem	Good child who does not contend with others; self-image easy to break down; average self-esteem
Personality	Cheerful, active; extroverted; independent; competitive	Shy, passive; introverted; dependent; noncompetitive
Precipitating factors	Conflicts with others; loss of peers' approval	Lowered school marks; loss of parents' approval
Psychotherapy	Change self-image; accept defeat, setbacks, weakness	Maintain self-image; verbalize inner negative feelings
Group experience	Accept being located in outer periphery	Experience being located in the center

Life History and Present History

The boy liked playing baseball beginning at primary school age and dreamed of someday being a professional baseball player. He joined the baseball club in the third grade of primary school. In secondary school he played on the baseball team, and he was a star player. He was also selected for a leading role in the student union. In high school he joined the baseball team, but baseball practice at this level was difficult and he began to have hyperventilation attacks in July. At the same time he had a low-grade fever and general fatigue, so he stopped practicing baseball. He was referred to several hospitals, but the cause of his illness was undetermined. In September he was thought to have tonsillitis and underwent a tonsillectomy. After the operation his low-grade fever disappeared temporarily, and he started baseball practice again. He was bullied at baseball practice by senior members and began to have a low-grade fever again. In December he was admitted to the Department of Otorhinolaryngology and in February was referred to the Department of Neuropsychiatry.

Clinical Course After Admission

Soon after admission he began to complain of a number of minor somatic symptoms, such as loss of appetite, headache, neck pain, and eye pain. Physical examinations were all normal. The nursing staff responded to his complaints inconsistently, and he began to accuse some of the nurses and doctors about having a poor attitude toward him. One month after admission, he complained of muscle weakness of the lower limbs and of being unable to walk. He also complained of sensory disturbance and muscle weakness of the right arm. He used a wheelchair in the unit. His management was discussed repeatedly at staff meetings. We decided to listen to his complaints, take his symptoms at face value, and introduce him to physical rehabilitation. He recovered gradually, and in May he was discharged to his home. At the time of discharge, he could walk but he still complained of mild muscle weakness of the lower limbs.

Clinical Course After Discharge

Soon after discharge he left the baseball team of the high school and joined a less competitive baseball club. After earning a star position in the club, his somatic symptoms disappeared completely. At the follow-up at age 19 he was doing well without symptoms.

Summary

This patient had a self-image that he was a completely "right," "strong," and "excellent" person, so he could not accept his setback in the competition of the baseball club. During individual psychotherapy one of the focuses was to get him to accept this setback. He insisted on continuing activity in the baseball club at first, but gradually he could accept changing his membership to a less competitive club. Through individual psychotherapy he was able to change his self-image somewhat. At last, by getting a star position in the less competitive club, his new self-image was supported.

Common Features of the Active Type

Parents of these patients describe their children as easy to raise and apparently independent of their parents during their infantile and childhood periods. They are looked on as reliable persons by their peers in primary and secondary school. In peer relationships they are socially well integrated into the group and take a leading role, such as that of a captain. Their self-image is that of an excellent person, and their self-esteem is high. Their personality is active, extroverted, and competitive. They are strong enough to contend with others, and they win frequently. They think that they have to be cooperative; but on the other hand, they cannot permit others' dishonesty. They therefore have a tendency to have conflicts, but they cannot sufficiently express their feelings verbally. Isolation in their peer relationships or lowered school marks threaten their self-image and high self-esteem, and precipitate conversion symptoms. Concerning psychotherapy, it is important for them to come to terms with their defeats, setbacks, and weaknesses. It is necessary for changes to occur in their self-image and self-esteem.

Passive Type of Conversion Disorders (Patients 13–18)

Patient 13

Patient 13, an 18-year-old girl, exemplifies the passive type of conversion disorder. There was nothing specific in her medical history, and her personality was quiet, modest, and timid. In her peer group she was a listener and follower. She tuned in to others' opinions and did not assert her own.

Family Background

Her father had an alcohol dependence, and her mother had anxiety disorders. The father became violent toward the mother and the girl after drinking too much. Her mother was a serious, introverted, asocial person. Both the mother and the patient feared the father and were mutually dependent on each other.

Life History and Present History

The subject was an obedient, compliant child who never opposed her parents' opinions. Her dream was to be a kindergarten or primary school teacher.

She sometimes complained of abdominal pain beginning in the first grade of high school. After her school marks fell in the third grade, she complained of eye pain and dizziness. In June she was admitted to the Department of Otorhinolaryngology. Her physical examinations were all normal, and she was referred to the Department of Neurology. From that time she began to have hyperventilation attacks and gait disturbance, and she also exhibited acting out behavior, such as running away from the ward. She was then referred and admitted to the Department of Neuropsychiatry.

Clinical Course After Admission

After admission she ran away again. She seemed self-centered and childish. Her ability to verbalize inner feelings was poor, and she acted out easily when she was frustrated. She exhibited hyperventilation, astasia, and abasia repeatedly in the ward. As a result of having limits set, she began to act out less frequently and be interested in her individual psychotherapy, which focused on supporting her self-image and verbalizing her feelings. Her somatic symptoms gradually disappeared through both individual and family psychotherapy.

After admission of the patient the mother became more anxious, and she asked for psychiatric treatment for herself. In individual psychotherapy she gradually gained insights that she was too dependent on her daughter and avoided her husband because of fear. She then began to think about her marital problems.

The father at first denied his alcoholism but gradually admitted it and its influence on his daughter and wife. He then joined an alcoholism recovery support group.

Clinical Course After Discharge

The patient graduated from high school and entered a small and less competitive business school. She became a scholarship student in the business school, and her symptoms disappeared completely after entering the school. She was doing well at age 24 at the time of follow-up.

Summary

The illness was precipitated by falling school marks and family problems. For her the crisis was precipitated by losing her good self-image. It seemed that her self-image had to be supported by individual psychotherapy and milieu manipulation. Work within the family group was also needed. The other focus of individual psychotherapy was on verbalizing her feelings. Recovery was finally achieved by gaining the approval of other students and teachers in the business school.

Common Features of the Passive Type

Parents of these patients describe their offspring as easy to raise and apparently obedient. The patients themselves are looked on as childish by their parents and their peers. In peer relationships, they are at the periphery of their groups, being followers and listeners. Their personality is quiet, introverted, noncompetitive, and passive. They do not express their negative feelings and are not even conscious of them. They avoid contending with others. Their self-image and self-esteem are not high and are easily broken down. Such self-image and self-esteem are barely sustained by their parents' approval, which is attained by the patients being obedient and compliant. They have a tendency to depend on significant others, especially their mothers. Loss of approval of these significant others threatens their self-image and self-esteem and precipitates conversion symptoms. Concerning psychotherapy it is important for these patients to obtain the approval of significant others—that means they can support their own self-images by the approval of others, so they must win it.

Discussion

Self-Image and Self-Esteem

Andrews [11] described the self-concept of the hysterical person as a pleasing person, one who is lovable, cooperative, and socially acceptable. He described how hostile or otherwise socially unacceptable feeling is excluded or suppressed from the hysteric's self-concept. This study also reveals the self-image of each of the patients as a "good" child. However, it is important to note that the meaning of "good" is different for the active type and the passive type person. "Good" to the active type person means someone who is superior to others, whereas to the passive type person it means someone who does not contend with others and who does not assert his or her opinions. The self-image of the active type is relatively stable, whereas the self-image of the passive type is fragile and easily disturbed. Self-images of both type are different each other but both need the others' evaluation and acknowledgement to be sustained.

Coleman [12] pointed out that self-esteem was closely related to general social adjustment and to the stability of the self-concept. He wrote that the higher the individual's self-esteem the better adjusted and the more stable in terms of self-concept he or she is likely to be. This study revealed that the active type has high self-esteem, high social adjustment, and stable self-image; and the passive type has average self-esteem, average social adjustment, and fragile self-image. My report is therefore consistent with that of Coleman [12]. Brown [13] divided peers into three categories according to their self-perceived relation to crowds: (1) crowd members (leaders or definite members of one crowd); (2) marginal members (those who have friends from different crowds but do not fit into any single group, or who are sometimes accepted by a group and sometimes not); (3) nonmembers (those who are loners or who have a couple of friends but do not fit into any crowd). I believe that the "active type" can be included in Brown's group 1 (crowd members) and the "passive type" has strong similarities with Brown's group 2 (marginal members).

Precipitating Factors and Formation of Hysterical Symptoms

Maloney [14] reported recent family stress and family communication problems, and Volkmar et al. [15] reported sexual stressors in 21 of 30 conversion disorders. Lehmkuhl et al. [4] reported employment of the mother (32%), academic failure (31%), peer conflicts (30%), and loss of a related person (29%) as abnormal psychosocial situations.

The present study reveals peer problems (eight patients), lowered school marks (five patients), and failure in a club or job (three patients) to be precipitating factors.

I believe that these precipitating factors threaten the self-image and self-esteem of patients. During their infancy and childhood they had few experiences that threatened their self-image of being a "good" child. During these periods they succeeded in maintaining their self-image of "good" child by suppressing and denying "bad" feelings and wishes that contradicted their self-image of "good" child. During adolescence, however, they had serious experiences, such as isolation from peers, lowered school marks, failure in a club activity, and so on. At the time they had "bad" feelings, such as hate, and "bad" wishes, such as a wish to escape from real life. For example, patient 1 wanted to leave her club activity and leave school, patient 10 wanted to quit her job, and patient 13 wanted to escape from school. Because these "bad" feelings and desires contradicted their self-image of "good" child, the feelings were suppressed and denied, and conversion symptoms and dissociative symptoms were formed.

These hysterical symptoms have several meanings. First, the symptoms express the patients' suppressed unconscious feelings and wishes. Second, the patients seek love and help from important others through their symptoms. Third, they can maintain their self-image of "good" child because they are "sick" and so cannot do what is expected of them. Therapists are needed to clarify these meanings for the patient.

Continuance and Worsening of Hysterical Symptoms

A secondary gain was found among these patients in that by their hysterical symptoms patients could escape from real life and attract love and attention from important others. This factor was important in the continuance of hysterical symptoms.

The hysterical symptoms of some patients (e.g., nos. 1, 7, 13, 17) worsened after they were referred to the hospital. This change occurred because their symptoms were explained insufficiently and inadequately. Sometimes their symptoms were explained by the staff as "psychogenic," "nothing wrong," or "mental disease," without concern for their psychological aspects.

As a result of these explanations the patients believed that their symptoms were not recognized as "real disease" or that their symptoms were suspected to be "pretended illness" or "factitious illness." These changes and the loss of others' positive evaluations and acknowledgment threatened their self-image of being a "good" child and caused worsening hysterical symptoms. I call these changes and loss "secondary loss." I believe that continuance and the worsening of hysterical symptoms during adolescence are more strongly influenced by "secondary loss" than "secondary gain." The patients continue to be ill not because they *can* attract love and attention from important others but because they *cannot*.

Alleviation of Hysterical Symptoms

Environmental factors related to improvement included joining a new group (especially a small, less competitive group) and acquiring friends of the opposite sex. In small, less competitive groups patients of the active type can regain a central position among their peers and regain the esteem and acknowledgment of important others. These factors enable the patients to recover their self-image of being a "good" child and their self-esteem. In small, less competitive groups, some patients of the passive type (nos. 13, 14) can attain a central position among their peers for the first time. This change from the outer periphery to a central position among their peers enables them to have a new self-image.

For some patients of the active type (nos. 6, 8) joining a new group enables them to come to terms with their previous defeat and setback by accepting the values of the new group and accepting a position on the outer periphery among peers.

Treatment

Several studies have reported the importance of limiting investigations to an essential minimum [4, 16–19] and promoting physical rehabilitation [4, 18, 19]. Collaboration between the physician and the psychiatrist from an early point is also important [18, 19]. I believe it is important to combine individual psychotherapy, physiotherapy, and milieu manipulation.

During individual psychotherapy, I approved of the efforts by active type patients to maintain the self-image of being a "good" child and in passive type patients to keep tuning into others' ideas and opinions. I then tried to change the self-image and self-esteem of the active type patients or to support or restore self-image and self-esteem in the passive type patients. One of the foci of individual psychotherapy for active type patients is to come to terms with defeat and setback and for passive type individuals to verbalize negative feelings. For the active type patient it is important to know that their real self, which may not be excellent, is approved by the therapist or significant others. For the passive type patient it is important to know that they have not been abandoned by the therapist or significant others even though they express negative feelings. It is also important for active type patients to accept not being in the central position in their peer group, whereas passive type patients benefit from the experience of being in a central position.

It is important for the therapist to establish a therapeutic milieu with parents and teachers. The therapist must advise parents and teachers to look at the patient's symptoms from their positive aspects (e.g., that they are the result of their efforts and predicaments) instead of the negative aspects (e.g., that they are an "escape into the illness"). This advice enables the patients to obtain positive approval, and positive approval enables the patients to "escape with honor" [18] from the symptoms. Approval by the peer group is especially important.

Follow-up

Robins and O'Neal [20] reported the follow-up of 23 patients and found that their prognoses were relatively poor. Proctor [21] reported that 15 of 25 patients recovered during hospitalization or soon after discharge. Slater and Glithero [22] pointed out that 33% of patients, originally diagnosed as suffering from hysteria, were later found to be suffering from organic disease. Caplan [23] also reported that 46% of patients originally diagnosed as suffering from hysteria during childhood and adolescence were found, on discharge or at follow-up, to have an organic basis. Rivinus et al. [24] reported 12 children with complaints that had been diagnosed as being due to a psychiatric disorder presented to a pediatric neurological unit, where neurological disease was diagnosed.

If the exclusion diagnosis is done precisely, the prognosis for the patient with a conversion disorder is relatively good. Caplan [23] reported that "true hysterics" showed both good recovery from their initial presenting symptoms 9–24 months later and good emotional adjustment at follow-up after 4–11 years. Leslie [19] reported that 17 of 20 children recovered completely within 3 months of starting treatment. This study revealed that conversion symptoms of five patients (27.8%) disappeared rapidly, in five patients (27.8%) they disappeared at 1–2 years, and in eight patients (44.4%) the conversion disorder continued for more than 2 years. Organic diseases were not found at follow-up. One of the reasons for this result is that in the Department of Neuropsychiatry first referral was soon followed by minimal neurological examination as well as psychotherapeutic work.

Cultural Aspects

Concerning the hysterical personality, several authors writing from psychoanalytical perspectives described two types of hysterical personality: One type is fixated at the phallic-genital level, and the other is fixated at the oral level [25]. The former type is better than the latter in terms of ego strength, superego structure, family background, peer relationships, social adaptation, and so on. The active type individual of the present study is almost congruent with the phalic-genital type and the passive type herein is almost congruent with the oral type. On some points, however, this result is different from those of Western studies. In terms of social adaptation, the orally fixated group has poor adaptation in Western countries, but the passive type in Japan had relatively good social adaptation both before and after treatment. Five of six patients adapted well at the time of follow-up. I believe that it is due to the cultural difference between Western countries and Japan. Dependence and passivity are more acceptable in Japanese society than in Western society, although the situation is changing. Sometimes a person who asserts opinions and negative feelings is more difficult to live with in a community than a person who asserts nothing. To be cooperative and not to assert opinions are still thought to be good manners in schools and companies. I believe that this situation helps the passive type individual to adapt in society more easily. Conversion disorders are closely related to the ability to verbalize, so this cultural difference may have a strong influence on symptom formation and social adaptation.

Conclusion

Eighteen adolescent patients (14 girls, 4 boys) with conversion disorders were studied. They were divided into three groups according to their personality characteristics, premorbid adaptation, and self-image. Group one (active type) was extroverted, active, and competitive and showed excellent adaptation. Group two (passive type) was introverted, passive, and noncompetitive and showed average adaptation. Group three had mixed characteristics. Self-image and self-esteem must be changed in the active type individual, whereas these traits need to be maintained and supported in the passive type person, through individual psychotherapy and milieu manipulation, including family counseling and group interactions.

This typification was done by personality characteristics, social adaptation, regard by others, self-image, and self-esteem, which were gained mainly from patients' and parents' descriptions. So, these methods have their limitations. The study suggests that such differentiation has some implications for treatment and outcome. Further refinement of our ability to distinguish these personality types could be useful.

References

1. Leff J (1988) Psychiatry around the globe. Gaskell, London
2. Goodyer I (1981) Hysterical conversion reactions in childhood. J Child Psychol Psychiatry 22: 179–188
3. Eggers C (1985) Hysterie im Kindesalter. Munch Med Wochenschr 127:422–427
4. Lehmkuhl G, Blanz B, Lehmkuhl U, Broun-Scharm H (1989) Conversion disorder (DSM-3 300.11): symptomatology and course in childhood and adolescence. Eur Arch Psychiatry Neurol Sci 238:155–160
5. Schecker NH (1987) Childhood conversion reactions in the emergency department. Part 1. Diagnostic and management approaches within a biopsychosocial framework. Pediatr Emerg Care 3:202–208
6. Steinhausen H, Aster M, Pfeiffer E, Gobel D (1989) Comparative study of conversion disorders in childhood and adolescence. J Child Psychol Psychiatry 30:615–621
7. Steinberg D (1987) Basic adolescent psychiatry. Blackwell, Oxford
8. Arakaki G (1963) On the chronological transition of concept of hysteria. Kyushu J Neuropsychiatry 10:71–95
9. Nishizono M (1980) Clinical study of hysteria (in Japanese). Jpn J Clin Psychiatry 9:1145–1156
10. Fukuda K, Moriyama M, Suzuki T (1980) Hysteria and urbanization. Br J Psychiatry 137:300–304
11. Andrews JDW (1984) Psychotherapy with the hysterical personality: an interpersonal approach. Psychiatry 47:211–232
12. Coleman J (1980) The nature of adolescence. Methuen, London
13. Brown BB (1986) The importance of peer group ("crowd") affiliation in adolescence. J Adolesc 9:73–96
14. Maloney MJ (1980) Diagnosis of hysterical conversion reactions in children. Pedatrics 97:1016–1020
15. Volkmar FR, Poll JP, Lewis M (1984) Conversion reactions in childhood and adolescence. J Am Acad Child Psychiatry 23:424–430
16. Rock NL (1971) Conversion reactions in childhood. J Am Acad Child Psychiatry 10:65–93
17. Friedman SB (1973) Conversion symptoms in adolescents. Pediatr Clin North Am 20:873–882
18. Dubowitz V, Hersov L (1976) Management of children with non-organic (hysterical) disorders of motor function. Dev Med Child Neurol 18:358–368
19. Leslie SA (1988) Diagnosis and treatment of hysterical conversion reactions. Arch Dis Child 63:506–511
20. Robins E, O'Neal P (1953) Clinical features of hysteria in children with a note on prognosis, a two to seventeen year follow-up study of 41 patients. Nerv Child 10:246–271
21. Proctor JT (1958) Hysteria in childhood. Am J Orthopsychiatry 28:394–407
22. Slater E, Glithero E (1965) A follow-up of patients diagnosed as suffering from "hysteria." J Psychosom Res 9:9–13
23. Caplan HL (1970) Hysterical "conversion" symptoms in childhood. M.Phil. dissertation, University of London
24. Rivinus TM, Lamison DL, Graham PJ (1975) Childhood organic neurological disease presenting as psychiatric disorder. Arch Dis Child 50:115–119
25. Lazare A (1971) The hysterical character in psychoanalytic theory. Arch Gen Psychiatry 25:131–137

Clinical Picture of Obsessive-Compulsive Disorder During Childhood

Yoshiki Ishisaka[1] and Yoshihiro Segawa[2]

Summary. Although childhood obsessive-compulsive disorder is not a clinically neg-ligible entity, few studies of the clinical picture and outcome of this illness have been reported. The present study was undertaken to investigate these aspects of the disor-der when it develops during childhood. The study subjects were 17 children who were examined and treated at the Psychiatry Clinic of the Kyoto University Hospital during the 6-year period between April 1981 and the end of March 1987. We obtained the following results: (1) The average age of disorder onset was 12.8 years. (2) Boys predominated, with the boy/girl ratio 4.67:1.00. (3) The temperament of the patients before onset was characterized as methodical in 11 patients and childish (immature) and selfish in 9. Seven patients had been cheerful and extroverted before disorder onset. More than half of all patients had neurotic habits. (4) Major symptoms were compulsive acts in 15 patients and obsessive ideas in 2 patients. (5) The outcome of treatment could be assessed in 16 patients. Symptoms disappeared completely in 5 patients and were reduced in the remaining 11. Nine patients were still receiving treatment at the time of outcome assessment. These results indicate the importance of helping patients with this disorder establish a sense of self, which enables them to lead a stable daily life after the disappearance of symptoms. Thus therapeutic efforts were not confined to the alleviation of symptoms.

Keywords. Obsessive-compulsive disorder—Clinical picture—Outcome—Childhood

Introduction

Obsession and compulsion are nonspecific mental phenomena. Various types of obsessions and compulsions can be seen, ranging from those related to normal ritual behaviors [1] and children's play [2] to those that accompany schizophrenia, depres-sion, and organic disorders [3]. Saltzman [1] suggested that obsessions sometimes underlie alcohol addiction, obesity, or thievish habits. Within this wide spectrum of obsessions, a generalized condition called obsessive-compulsive disorder comprises a

[1] Department of Psychiatry, Faculty of Medicine, Kyoto University, 53 Kawahara-cho, Shogoin, Sakyo-ku, Kyoto 606, Japan
[2] Kansai Child and Adolescent Sanatorium, 838 Nishiwaki, Iwaoka-cho, Nishi-ku, Kobe 674, Japan

major portion. This condition has attracted the close attention of clinicians for years, and numerous studies have been conducted.

It is known that obsessive-compulsive disorder is often first diagnosed or noted during the decade between 10 and 19 years of age. According to a survey of 57 cases by Mueller [4], two-thirds manifested this problem before age 20. Kringlen [5] found that half of the patients he examined had developed this disorder before age 20, and that about 20% of them developed it before age 15. In Japan, Yoshida [6] reported that about 40% of the patients he examined had developed this disorder between 10 and 19 years of age.

Matsumoto et al. [7] analyzed the age at onset of this disorder in detail and noted two age peaks at which this disorder developed, between 10 and 19 years. Based on this finding, they classified obsessive-compulsive disorder into adolescent and juvenile types. The percentage of patients with this disorder who developed it before age 15 is not negligible, although it varies among surveys: from 37% [8], to 20% [5, 9], to 8% [10].

Matsumoto et al. [7] suggested that the outcome is better for the juvenile type than for the adolescent type. The type of obsessive-compulsive disorder that develops during the ages corresponding to the age group called "juvenile" by Matsumoto et al. has not been adequately studied, although several investigators [2, 11–15] have reported studies about this type. We recently examined the outcome for the juvenile type of this condition, using the classification of Matsumoto et al. [7], and found that its outcome was considerably better than we had anticipated. Our findings as to the clinical picture of this type of obsessive-compulsive disorder, including its outcome, are presented here.

Definition

As stated above, the phenomena called obsession and compulsion accompany many psychiatric illnesses. To allow cases of obsessive-compulsive disorder to be distinguished from other cases with these symptoms, a clear definition of obsessive-compulsive disorder is necessary. The definition of this condition offered by Schneider [16, 17] is often referred to. According to his definition, obsessions are thoughts experienced as senseless, or at least unreasonably dominant, yet irresistible [17]. The definition of Saltzman [1] includes the presence of anxiety or physical discomfort associated with such thoughts. The definition of obsessions contained in the *DSM-III* [18] is almost the same as that of Schneider, except that the former additionally refers to disturbances of social function, an inability to fulfill one's social role, or embarrassment on the part of the individual because of having these thoughts. Disturbances of social function, referred to in the *DSM-III*, are caused by the disorder. Although it may be important to emphasize such disturbances when treating this condition, they are useless for defining obsessive-compulsive disorder. The definition contained in the *ICD-9* [19] is close to the definition of Salzman and was the one used for making judgments of obsessive-compulsive disorder in the present study.

Subjects and Methods

The subjects were patients who satisfied the criteria for the diagnosis of obsessive-compulsive disorder contained in the *ICD-9* and who were first examined at less than 15 years of age at the Psychiatry Clinic of the Kyoto University Hospital during the 6-

year period between April 1981 and the end of March 1987. During the same 6-year period, 413 patients younger than 15 years were first examined at this clinic. The medical records, obtained at our clinic, showed a diagnosis of obsessive-compulsive disorder in 24 of the 413 patients; 7 of these 24 patients did not receive treatment at our clinic after the first examination because (1) they discontinued visiting the clinic or (2) they were referred to other facilities for various reasons. After excluding these 7 patients, 17 remained and were included in the present study. For these 17 subjects, we analyzed the age at the onset of the disorder, their temperament before disorder onset, family profiles, apparent prodromal signs, precipitating factors, symptoms, course of treatment, and the outcome of treatment. For patients who were still being treated at the time of outcome assessment, we assessed them directly in the clinical setting. For those were not patients at the time of outcome assessment, a questionnaire was sent to their family. Using these methods, the outcome of treatment could be assessed for all but one patient. The data collected by this survey can be therefore regarded as fairly reliable concerning the outcome of our subjects. The assessment of outcome was based on the evaluation of two factors—changes in symptoms and social adaptation—according to the method of Grimshaw [20].

Results

Table 1 shows the subjects' ages at first examination, estimated age at onset, sex, family profiles, temperament before onset, prodromal signs, precipitating factors, major symptoms, brief course of treatment, length of time from the first examination to the survey, and the patient's state at the time of the survey.

Boys predominated, with a male/female ratio of 4.67:1.00 (Table 2). The average age of onset of the disorder was 12.8 years and the average age at the first examination 13.3 years. Table 3 shows that the most frequent age of onset was 13 years (five cases), followed by 12 years (four cases) and 14 years (three cases). These results suggest that obsessive-compulsive disorder is likely to develop at 12 to 14 years of age (most frequently at 13 years). The lowest age of onset among this population was 9 years.

Our survey of family profiles revealed that five fathers and three mothers were methodical, and three fathers and four mothers were nervous. Furthermore, two fathers were strict disciplinarians, and one mother had great anxiety. One mother had epilepsy, but no other parent had evident psychiatric disorder.

The analysis of the patients' temperament revealed that 11 patients were methodical, and 9 were childish and selfish (the numbers of patients include some duplications). Four patients tended to be gloomy and introverted. It is noteworthy that seven patients were cheerful and extroverted (Table 4).

Prodromal signs observed include tic (three cases), nail biting (five cases), and bed wetting (two cases) (Table 5). Of the 17 patients, 8 had some signs that could be psychiatrically regarded as prodromal signs. Neurotic habits were noted in more than half of all subjects. Events that seem to have triggered the onset of disorder were identified in 7 (41%) of the 17 patients. For three patients, the experience of being bullied at school seemed to have served as a precipitating factor. Failure to pass the junior high school entrance examination seemed to have served this purpose in one case and a change of school venue seemed to have triggered the onset in another. These results suggest that mental trauma related to school often triggers the onset of this disorder in children of this age group.

Table 1. Patients and their clinical characteristics.

Sex	Age at onset/age at first exam	Family profile	Temperament	Precursing signs	Precipitating factor	Symptoms	Course	Follow-up after first exam (years: months)	Outcome
M	9:8/9:11	Father: self employed, methodical, strict in discipline Mother: methodical, nervous Brother: 4 years older	Cheerful, many friends		Surgery for inguinal hernia	Repetition of walk, object-holding	Symptoms disappeared after 3 months hospital stay and 1 year treatment	4:5	Symptoms disappeared. No problem in daily life. Attending school. Cured.
M	9:10/10:0	Father: employee, nervous Mother: kimono dyeing specialist, nervous Sister: 5 years younger	Tenacious, fastidious	Bed-wetting (until the third year of elementary school) nail biting, thumb sucking (began recently)	Anxiety caused by being told some curse words by a friend	Repetition of particular actions, slow motion, repetition of saying "sorry"	Symptoms disappeared after 1 year of ambulatory treatment	2:3	Symptoms disappeared. No problem in daily life. Attending school. Cured.
M	10:5/12:11	Father: employee, taciturn, timid Mother: talkative, anxious Sister: 3 years younger	Methodical, cheerful, tenacious			Repetition of actions, frequent hand washing, shouting loudly, repetition of the same words, fickleness	Symptoms reduced slightly by 2 years of ambulatory treatment, but visit discontinued thereafter		Unknown.
M	11:6/13:3	Father: self-employed, nervous, gentle Mother: optimist Sister: 4 years younger	Methodical, introverted, selfish		Bullied at school	Frequent hand washing, slow motion, abusive language, tic	Being treated after first examined 5 years ago (including 1 year hospital stay)	5:7	Symptoms disappeared almost completely. No problem in daily life. Working. Almost cured.
M	11:8/12:0	Father: self-employed Mother: nurse, irritable Sister: 3 years younger	Methodical, selfish	Tic (in the third year of elementary school)		Fixation on certain letters in a book; obsession with dirt on books (cannot help but cutting out the dirty portion)	One month stay at our hospital and later referred to another hospital where he is now being treated as an outpatient	3:10	Tendency to become anxious remains. Frequently blows his nose. School life possible. Slightly improved.
F	12:2/14:1	Father: merchant Mother: private school teacher Sister: 3 years younger	Cheerful in the past, but introverted since entering junior high school	Hyperreaction to fearful story during elementary school	Change of school	Repetition of actions (writing and immediately erasing letters, apologizing for God)	Receiving ambulatory treatment	3:0	Symptoms of obsession have disappeared almost completely. Difficulty with personal relationships. Tends to be emotionally unstable. Sometimes absent from school.

Table 1. *Continued.*

Sex	Age at onset/age at first exam[a]	Family profile	Temperament	Precursing signs	Precipitating factor	Symptoms	Course	Follow-up after first exam (years: months)	Outcome
M	12:4/13:6	Father: self-employed, nervous, quiet. Mother: methodical, strong-minded, fastidious. Sister: 2 years older, active	Methodical, introverted, short-tempered			Frequent hand washing; remaining in his own room, saying his mother and elder sister are dirty	Resumed school life after 2.5 years of treatment (including 1.5 years of hospital stay)	3:0	Feeling that his mother is dirty is sometimes seen, but no problem in daily life. Attending school. Improved.
M	12:6/12:9	Father: Noh player. Mother: Brother: 2 years older. Sister: 2 years younger	Nervous, methodical	Nail biting (during elementary school), playing with genitals		Anxious about mathematics, anxious because he feels he may have injured others	Symptoms subsided after 1 month of ambulatory treatment	5:6	Symptoms disappeared. No problem in daily life. Attending school. Cured.
M	12:7/12:11	Father: teacher. Mother: teacher, dependent on others. Brothers: younger brother died soon after birth; another brother 3 years younger	Methodical, nervous, selfish		Failure in junior high school entrance examination	Obsession with arranging objects, habit of checking, slow motion	Hospitalized twice because of violence against family and tendency to remain in his own room	8:6	Symptoms reduced but have not disappeared completely. No problem in daily life. Improved.
M	13:3/13:5	Father: public official, strict in discipline. Mother: nonchalant. Brother: 2 years younger. Grandmother/great grandmother:	Cheerful, quiet, selfish		Bullied at school	Frequent hand washing, dirt phobia, tends to remain in his own room	Symptoms disappeared after treatment (including 1 year of hospital stay)	4:5	Some symptoms persist. Bathes 2–4 times a day. Slow in making a decision. Attending school. Slightly improved.
F	13:8/14:0	Father: public official, methodical. Mother: Sister: 6 years younger	Cheerful, anxious about her reputation, childish	Bed-wetting (until second year of elementary school), nail biting (until the fourth year of elementary school), enuresis (fifth year of elementary school)	Separated from grandmother; bullied at school	Frequent hand washing, dirt phobia, tic, stammering, violence against family	Continues to receive treatment (including 3 months of hospital stay in the past)	1:5	Compulsive act and tic have been reduced. Attending school although irregularly. No problem in daily life. Improved.

Sex	Age	Family background	Personality	Past history	Symptoms	Treatment	Ratio	Outcome
M	13:10/14:10	Father: company executive, strict in discipline Mother: nervous Brother: 7 years younger	Cheerful, selfish, short-tempered		Frequent hand washing, dirt phobia, anxious about various matters	Hospitalized twice because of compulsive act, violence against family and attempted suicide; being treated as an outpatient	6:5	Anxiety during writing persists, but no problem in daily life. Slightly improved.
M	13:11/14:1	Father: employee, earnest, methodical, short-tempered Mother: Eldest sister: 4 years older 2nd Eldest sister: 2 years older Younger sister: 2 years younger	Methodical, introverted, quiet, anxious around others	Nail biting (until the sixth year of elementary school)	Frequent hand washing, anxious, frequent change of clothes	Symptoms disappeared after 1.5 years of ambulatory treatment	5:1	Symptoms disappeared. No problem in daily life. Gave up senior high school. Living at home.
F	13:11/13:11	Father: employee, methodical, earnest Mother: earnest Brother: 2 years younger.	Short-tempered, selfish, quiet, methodical	Nail biting (until the sixth year of elementary school)	Frequent hand washing, dirt phobia, anxious about trivial matters	Symptoms disappeared after 1.5 years of treatment (including hospital stay); being treated as an outpatient	1:10	Symptoms reduced but remains anxious in daily life. Cannot attend school. Slightly improved.
M	14:6/14:7	Father: self-employed Mother: Brothers: 3 younger brothers (1, 3, and 6 years younger)	Introverted, selfish, timid		Frequent hand washing, dirt phobia	Symptoms disappeared after 3 visits to the outpatient clinic	5:11	Symptoms disappeared. No problem in daily life. Attending a university. Cured.
M	14:6/14:11	Father: company executive, methodical, nervous Mother: nervous Sister: 8 years older	Methodical, timid, quiet		Thinking about various matters and anxious about them, frequently stops breathing intentionally	Symptoms disappeared after 2 months of ambulatory treatment	2:10	Symptoms disappeared. No problem in daily life. Attending school. Cured.

*9:8, nine years eight months.

Table 2. Male/female ratio, mean age of onset, and mean age at first examination.

Male/female ratio	4.67:1.00
Age of onset	12.8 years
Age at first examination	13.3 years

Table 3. Distribution of age of onset and symptoms.

Age (years)	Compulsive behavior		Obsessive ideas		Total
	Male	Female	Male	Female	
9	2				2
10	1				1
11	2				2
12	2	1	1		4
13	3	2			5
14	2		1		3
Total	12	3	2		17

Table 4. Characteristics of the temperaments of patients.

Characteristic	No. of patients[a]
Methodical	11
Childish, selfish	9
Cheerful, extroverted	7
Gloomy, introverted	4

[a] Numbers include some duplications.

Table 5. Prodromal symptoms.

Symptom	No. of patients[a]
Nail biting, thumb sucking	5
Tic	3
Bed wetting	2
Playing with genitals	1
Hyperreaction to fearful stories	1

[a] Numbers include some duplications.

Table 6 summarizes the major symptoms observed in the patients. Frequent hand-washing and dirt phobia were marked in eight patients, and other repetitive behaviors were seen in five. There were only two patients in whom obsessive ideas were major symptoms. Thus major symptoms of obsessive-compulsive disorder in this age group were compulsive acts rather than obsessive ideas. Table 3 analyzes the age of disorder onset for those patients in whom obsessive ideas or compulsive acts were marked.

When the period of treatment was analyzed, some patients no longer required treatment after only 1 month, whereas some patients continued to receive outpatient treatment 3 to 4 years after the start of treatment. Because of such great interindividual variation, it was not possible to calculate the average time from the start to the end of treatment.

Table 6. Major symptoms.

Symptom	No. of patients
Handwashing, dirt phobia	8
Repetitive behavior	5
Object arrangement	1
Breath holding	1
Fixation on certain letters/numbers	2

Of the 17 patients, 7 underwent outpatient treatment alone, and 10 were hospitalized. The fact that about 60% of all patients could not be appropriately treated as outpatients and required hospitalization indicates the importance of the symptoms when managing patients with this type of disorder. There were two factors that indicated hospitalization was required: (1) patients were unable to visit outpatient clinics because they remained in their rooms; and (2) patient care at home was difficult because the patient used violence against the family or the family was caught up in the patient's obsessive symptoms.

Outpatient treatment primarily comprised interviews between the psychiatrist and the patient, although interviews between the psychiatrist and the patient's family were conducted when necessary. During the psychiatrist–patient interviews the patients were encourage to talk about and describe their symptoms and express any underlying feelings of anxiety. At the same time, the psychiatrist gave the patients information about obsessive symptoms. In this way, the psychiatrist attempted to establish a therapeutic relationship while expressing sympathy with the patients because of their anxiety.

They also advised the patients about trying to refrain from compulsive acts. It is not possible for patients to stop all their compulsive acts at once. For this reason, during the course of treatment we focused on the compulsive acts that seemed easier to discontinue or to decrease in degree. The psychiatrist thus advised the patients to stop performing selected compulsive acts. At the next interview the psychiatrist asked if the target acts had been stopped. If the patients had followed the advice even slightly, the psychiatrist praised their efforts and set a new target. It is difficult for children in this age group to express their thoughts or feelings verbally. For this reason, we thought it better to focus the treatment of these children on advice about daily behaviors. At the same time, we attempted verbally to convince the patients of their safety in order to reduce any anxiety that might arise when they stopped performing the compulsive acts.

For inpatients, we first established a therapeutic relationship with each individual. Then, while the patient was performing their compulsive acts the psychiatrist verbally instructed the patient to stop. Sometimes the psychiatrist compelled the patient to stop, but even in these cases, the psychiatrist made efforts to guide the patient to stop the acts in several steps. The anxiety that arose in the patients following discontinuation of the compulsive acts was relieved by verbal assurance of their safety. In brief, it was necessary for the psychiatrist involved in the treatment of inpatients to support them so they could overcome any anxiety that arose after the compulsive acts were discontinued. This step is necessary because coping with the anxiety that underlies symptoms is essential to the treatment of this disorder.

The average length of follow-up of the patients treated in this way was 4.1 years from the first examination. Table 7 shows the outcome of treatment. Symptoms

Table 7. Outcome.

Outcome	No. of patients
Signs	
Disappeared completely	5
Reduced	11
Unchanged	0
Worsened	0
Social adaptation	
School or occupation resumed	10
Staying at home but no problem in daily life	6
Difficulty in daily life	0

disappeared completely in 5 patients and were reduced in the other 11. When social adaptation was assessed, 10 patients showed good adaptation and resumed attending school or their occupation, and 6 had no problem dealing with their daily lives, although they remained at home. Thus the symptoms of all patients completely disappeared or were reduced.

Discussion

It is well known that obsessive phenomena are seen at a fairly early stage of child development in the forms of play or rituals [2, 21]. At what age does the pathologic form of obsessive-compulsive disorder begin to be seen? Adams [2] reported cases of this disorder that developed at age 4. The average age of onset was 5.84 years for the 49 patients he examined. When we read his case reports, however, it is doubtful that we would diagnose obsessive-compulsive disorder for the patients in whom he reported the disorder to develop at age 4 or 6. Judd [11] described a case that developed at 6 years 4 months. Koelker [12] reported a patient in whom the disorder developed at age 5 years 4 months. In Japan, Wakabayashi [13] noted a patient in whom the disorder developed at age 5 years 2 months. The youngest age of onset of this disorder in our population was 9 years 8 months. At that age a diagnosis of obsessive-compulsive disorder is not uncommon. Thus although obsessive-compulsive disorder can develop even at around age 5, the disorder is rare at that age and it seems to develop primarily after age 10.

Regarding the temperaments of patients with obsessive-compulsive disorder, Wakabayashi [13] listed the following neurotic temperaments: earnest, methodical, perfectionistic, fearful, timid, careful, anxious, introverted, passive, dependent, and short-tempered. Apter et al. [22] noted obsessive personalities in three of the eight patients they examined. Rosenberg [23] reported that adults with obsessive-compulsive disorder have an obsessive personality, childishness, and a schizoid character. Some investigators have pointed out that patients with this disorder tend to be hyperreactive and obsessive in character [24]. Of the patients we studied, 9 tended to be childish and self-centered and 11 to be obsessive in character. However, because seven of our patients were cheerful and extroverted, we must point out that the temperament of patients with obsessive-compulsive disorder is not always neurotic. Based on these findings, we can roughly classify the preonset temperament of children with obsessive-compulsive disorder as obsessive and immature types. At the same time, we must bear in mind that the temperament of some children before the onset of this disorder is cheerful or extroverted and appears to have no relation to their later compulsive symptoms.

Other than these features of the temperament of children with this disorder, it is noteworthy that more than half of the patients we examined had had neurotic habits (e.g., tic, nail biting, bed wetting) before the onset of disorder, and that in 45% some factor seemed to have triggered the onset of the disorder. These precipitating factors were often related to school events. Wakabayashi also reported that the precipitating factors were related to school and learning for 80% of the patients he examined. If these results are considered together, it appears that the onset of obsessive-compulsive disorder after about 10 years of age can be explained by the inability of children with hyperreactive or obsessive tendencies to adapt to social demands and the resultant neurotic course, although these children had been able to adapt to the real world before disorder onset despite the presence of neurotic habits.

That the family members of patients with obsessive-compulsive disorder also had psychiatric abnormalities has been reported for years. A similar trend is seen with childhood obsessive-compulsive disorder. Hall, whose report of two cases of this disorder in 1935 was the earliest published account [25], and Despert [26], who reported four cases of this disorder, found that at least one of the parents of each of the patients was mentally abnormal in some way. Adams [2] reported that 71.4% of the families of the patients he examined had obsessive-compulsive disorder, and that 55% of the families had other psychiatric abnormalities. Hollingsworth et al. [27] reported that 82% of the families of 17 patients had severe physical disorder or psychiatric abnormalities, and seven mothers and four fathers showed marked obsessive tendencies.

In contrast, some investigators have reported that families of patients showed no marked differences in the prevalence of obsessive-compulsive disorder compared with the control families, although the prevalence of depression and alcoholism was higher in the families of patients [8]. Others have reported that no characteristic psychiatric abnormalities were detected in the parents of patients [28].

Wakabayashi [14] reported that 68% of the patients seemed to have been greatly affected during the course of personality development by some family member (e.g., a parent) who had an obsessive tendency. When we examined the parents of our 17 patients, there were eight fathers and seven mothers who were nervous or methodical in character, but no family member had evident psychiatric abnormalities. At the time of our survey, we detected no psychiatric abnormalities in any siblings of our patients. In view of these results, it seems unlikely that the prevalence of evident psychiatric abnormalities is higher among the parents of patients with obsessive-compulsive disorder than among control families, although the parents of patients did tend to be more frequently methodical, obsessive, or anxious.

Of the 17 patients we examined, 15 performed marked compulsive acts (Table 6), such as repetitive hand washing or other repetitive actions, and only two patients had obsessive ideas as a major symptom.

Matsumoto et al. [7] detected two peaks for the age of onset of obsessive-compulsive disorder during adolescence and categorized these cases as juvenile or adolescent. According to their report, the major symptom is compulsive acts for the juvenile type and obsessive ideas for the adolescent type. Compulsive acts were the major symptom in patients under 15 years of age.

Wakabayashi [14] reported a similar finding, which may be explained as follows. During the first half of the decade ages 10 to 19, children are not usually mentally mature enough to deal with their feelings of uncertainty or anxiety at the level of ideas or to form symptoms corresponding to their feelings. For this reason, children at this stage of development are obliged to take direct actions to cope with their feelings of uncertainty or anxiety, instead of dealing with them at the level of ideas. It may also explain why children with this disorder often answer "I don't know" or "I couldn't help doing it" when they are questioned after their symptoms have disappeared as to the reason why they manifested such obsessive symptoms.

Narita et al. [24] classified adult obsessive-compulsive disorder as a self-contained type and an "others-involving" type, saying that the latter type is more characteristic of women in whom the disorder developed during adulthood. Our patients with this disorder were alternately dependent on or controlling of their family members (especially their mothers) and tended to manipulate their family members (chiefly the mother). When the attempt to control the mother in this way failed, these children tended to demonstrate panic.

Such a tendency was also referred to by Judd [11]. The involvement of family members in the symptoms of this disorder was noted in five of the eight patients examined by Apter et al. [22] and in all of the 15 patients examined by Bolton et al. [29]. Koelker [12] emphasized the absolute monarch-like aspect of children with obsessive-compulsive disorder.

This tendency of children with the disorder seems to represent their attempt to reduce their anxiety by depending on surrounding people to solve problems because they cannot deal with their anxiety by themselves owing to the immaturity of their personalities. The information concerning the involvement of others in the patient's symptoms is important when selecting a method of treatment for this disorder. In 10 of the 17 patients we examined, the families were involved in the patients' symptoms, making outpatient treatment difficult for them and so requiring hospitalization.

Obsessive-compulsive disorder has been variously described to be a severe disorder [3] and, paradoxically, to have a poor outcome in some cases and relatively easy recovery in others [30]. To date, several surveys of the outcome of treatment for adults with this disorder have been reported. Taschev [10] found that of the 467 patients with *zwangskranheit* 38 recovered and 362 improved. His findings suggest that this disorder has a relatively good outcome. Mueller [4, 31] reported that the disorder disappeared or was reduced markedly in 28 of their 57 cases. Another report [25] indicated a similar response rate (recovery or reduction of symptoms in 40%). According to one report [9], 71% of 88 cases showed recovery or marked reduction, whereas another study [5] found that the percentage of patients showing recovery or marked reduction during a 30-year follow-up period on average after onset was only 9%.

On the basis of these studies, it seems that adults' obsessive-compulsive disorder responds better to treatment than it had been previously thought. The disorder still presents many difficulties before a cure is possible. However, Yoshida [6] reported that 16 (43%) of the 37 patients in whom this disorder had developed more than 5 years before responded to treatment, and Inagaki [32] reported that the symptoms of a patient with this disorder disappeared following psychological therapy 30 years after its onset at age 10. Hence it seems likely that this disorder can be cured even many years after its onset.

Regarding the outcome of this disorder in children, Berman [33] reported six cases and found that although symptoms disappeared rapidly the long-term outcome was poor because of a high incidence of schizophrenia or chronic disorder. The two patients examined by Hall [25] were reported to have repeated cycles of improvement and exacerbation. Bolton et al. [29] followed 13 patients and confirmed recovery in 7. Hollingsworth et al. [27] followed 10 patients for an average of 6.5 years and reported that symptoms disappeared completely in three and were reduced in seven.

Wakabayashi [15] conducted a long-term follow-up study in 14 patients: six (43%) showed complete disappearance of symptoms and good social adaptation, two continued to have obsessive symptoms after the end of treatment, one had anxiety disorder, and one was delusional. All of these patients could adapt themselves to social demands, but two had some difficulty with this adaptation.

Of the 16 patients in our study for whom the outcome of treatment could be assessed, 5 had adapted to the demands of the society and showed no problems, and 11 had some obsessive symptoms but had no serious problems in their daily lives. There were no patients whose symptoms exacerbated or remained unchanged, although nine of the patients were still receiving treatment at the time of the survey. In other words, there were many patients who required some therapeutic intervention even after the disappearance or reduction of obsessive symptoms because they were likely to feel anxious or become hypersensitive during daily life.

According to past studies of this disorder in children, symptoms disappear temporarily in about half of the cases. As seen in our patients, the symptoms of some children with obsessive-compulsive disorder disappear or are markedly reduced. Some of these children can lead their daily lives without particular problems even when their initial state was severe enough to require hospitalization, whereas others require a considerable degree of therapeutic intervention even after reduction or disappearance of their symptoms. Our treatment was aimed at supporting the patients while they endured their background anxiety for some time and helping them to be able to cope with their problems of daily life without presenting obsessive symptoms. The patients learned to express their anxiety when facing problems in daily life, and in order to resolve the anxiety some of them had to receive treatment for long periods of time. Even when we take this condition into account, the treatment of obsessive-compulsive disorder in children should not be aimed solely at the symptoms; it should be aimed at guiding the patients to grow from being individuals with neurotic postures (i.e., obsessive symptoms) into individuals who can lead a stable daily life without using neurotic solutions. After patients have rid themselves of their obsessive-compulsive disorder, it seems necessary for the psychiatrist to continue therapeutic intervention and family guidance for a relatively long period so the patient's sense of self, which does not have adequate protection, can grow into becoming capable of coping with reality.

Our follow-up was for only 4.1 years on average. Therefore the outcome of this disorder for longer periods cannot be predicted by our study at present. We cannot rule out that symptoms may recur over the long term.

In the present study, we could not definitely identify factors that would affect the outcome for this disorder. In this respect, Negishi [34] reported that symptoms tended to disappear or be reduced more frequently in cases where the fundamental temperament had not been seriously biased, the onset of the disorder was at a later age, and symptoms were simple. When our cases were analyzed, symptoms were more likely to be alleviated in cases where the disorder developed at a young age, probably because the obsessive symptoms of these children appeared in response to the outer world in fairly undisguised forms and because correction of the outer world resulted in disappearance of these symptoms (cases 1 and 2). Therefore this disorder may be easier to treat in cases where obsessive symptoms are in fairly pure forms and the onset of the disorder is related to the external environment.

In any event, our survey of the outcome of treatment revealed that the symptoms of obsessive-compulsive disorder during childhood are much more likely to disappear or decrease than has been thought, if treatment is given. At the same time, the survey revealed that therapeutic intervention needs to be continued for fairly long periods after the disappearance of symptoms, so the patient can establish a stable sense of self.

Conclusion

Of the patients who were first examined at the Psychiatric Clinic of the Kyoto University Hospital over the 6-year period between April 1981 and March 1987, 24 patients younger than 15 years of age satisfied the *ICD-9* criteria for the diagnosis of obsessive-compulsive disorder. Of these 24 patients, 17 were treated at our clinic. Clinical features of obsessive-compulsive disorder of childhood were evaluated in these 17 patients. The following results were obtained.

1. The disorder often developed in the age range between 12 and 14 years, with a peak at 13 years. The average age of disorder onset was 12.8 years.

2. Boys predominated, with the male/female ratio being 4.67:1.00.

3. The temperament of the patients before onset was characterized as methodical in 11 patients and childish (immature) and selfish in 9 (some children had two or more characteristics). Seven patients, however, had been cheerful and extroverted before disorder onset. More than half of all patients had neurotic habits, such as tic or bed wetting.

4. Family profiles revealed that eight fathers and seven mothers tended to be methodical, nervous, or anxious. No parents had evident psychiatric disorder.

5. Major symptoms were compulsive acts (e.g., frequent hand washing and repetitive behavior). There were two patients whom obsessive ideas were the major symptom.

6. The outcome of treatment could be assessed for 16 cases. Symptoms disappeared completely in 5 patients and were reduced in the other 11. Regarding social adaptation, 10 patients had resumed attending school or an occupation, and 6 patients remained at home although none of the six had problems with their daily activities at home. None of the 16 patients had any problems in daily life caused by symptoms of this disorder. This fact indicates that although obsessive-compulsive disorder during childhood is often severe enough to require hospitalization its symptoms are likely to disappear or decrease in response to treatment.

Nine patients had to continue treatment even after their symptoms disappeared or were reduced. It therefore seems important for the psychiatrist to help patients who have this disorder establish a sense of self, which enables them to lead a stable daily life, instead of confining therapeutic efforts to the alleviation of symptoms.

References

1. Salzman L (1975) The obsessive personality, origins, dynamics and therapy. Jason Aronson, New York
2. Adams P (1973) Obsessive children; a sociopsychiatric study. Brunner/Mazel, New York
3. Hirata K (1961) A consideration of obsessionals. Psychiatr Neurol Jpn 63:673–687

4. Mueller C (1957) Weitere Beobachtungen zum Verlauf der Zwangskrankheit. Psychiatr Neurol 133:80–94
5. Kringlen E (1965) Obsessional neurotics; a long-term follow-up. Br J Psychiatry 111:709–722
6. Yoshida M (1986) A clinical study of the prognosis of in tractable obsessive-compulsive neurosis. Jpn J Psychopathol 7:385–398
7. Matsumoto M, Ishizaka Y, Tamura Y, et al (1985) A clinical study of obsessive-compulsive neurosis in adolescence. Clin Psychiatry 27:1113–1122
8. Insel TR, Hoover C, Murphy DL (1983) Parents of patients with obsessive-compulsive disorder. Psychol Med 13:807–811
9. Lo WH (1967) A follow up study of obsessional neurosis in Hong Kong Chinese. Br J Psychiatry 113:823–832
10. Taschev T (1970) Zur Klinik der Zwangszustaende. Fortschr Neurol Psychiatry 38:89–110
11. Judd LE (1965) Obsessive compulsive neurosis in children. Arch Gen Psychiatry 12:136–143
12. Koelker U (1987) Zwangssyndrome im Kindes und Jugendalter. Vandenhoeck & Ruprecht, Goettingen
13. Wakabayashi S (1964) A study of childhood neurosis. J Nagoya Med Assoc 87:245–296
14. Wakabayashi S (1969) A consideration of the etiology of obsessive-compulsive neurosis in childhood. Bull Jap Univ Soc Welfare 16:173–200
15. Wakabayashi S (1980) The clinical course of a patient diagnosed as having obsessive-compulsive neurosis in childhood. Psychiatr Neurol Jpn 82:509–510
16. Schneider K (1923) Die Psychopathischen Persoenlichkeiten. Franz Deuticke, Vienna
17. Schneider K (1946) Klinische Psychopathologie. Georg Thieme, Stuttgart
18. American Psychiatric Association (1980) Diagnostic and statistic manual of mental disorders, 3rd edn. American Psychiatric Association, Washington, DC
19. World Health Organization (1978) Mental disorder glossary and guide to their classification in accordance with the ninth revision of the international classification of diseases. World Health Organization, Geneva
20. Grimshaw L (1965) The outcome of obsessional disorder; a follow-up study of 100 cases. Br J Psychiatry 111:1051–1056
21. Kanner L (1972) Child psychiatry, 4th edn. Charles C Thomas, Springfield, IL
22. Apter A, Bernhout E, Tyano S (1984) Severe obsessive compulsive disorder in adolescence; a report of eight cases. J Adolesc 7:349–358
23. Rosenberg CM (1967) Personality and obsessive neurosis. Br J Psychiatry 113:471–477
24. Narita Y, Nakamura U, Mizuno N, et al (1974) A consideration of obsessive-compulsive neurosis; self-confined type and others-involving type. Clin Psychiatry 16:957–964
25. Hall MB (1935) Obsessive-compulsive states in childhood and their treatment. Arch Dis Child 10:49–59
26. Despert JL (1968) Schizophrenia in children. Brunner/Mazel, New York
27. Hollingsworth CE, Tanguay PE, Grossman L, et al (1980) Long-term outcome of obsessive-compulsive disorder in childhood. J Am Acad Child Psychiatry 19:134–144
28. Rapoport J, Elkins R, Langer DH, et al (1981) Childhood obsessive-compulsive disorder. Am J Psychiatry 138:1545–1554
29. Bolton D, Collins S, Steinberg D (1983) The treatment of obsessive-compulsive disorder in adolescence; a report of fifteen cases. Br J Psychiatry 142:456–464
30. Nakagawa S (1954) Statistical and clinical studies on the prognosis of neuroasthenic-like state and obsessive-compulsive neurosis. Psychiatr Neurol Jpn 56:135–186
31. Mueller C (1953) Vorlaeufige Mitteilung zur langen Katamnese der Zwangskranken. Nervenarzt 24:112–115
32. Inagaki T (1982) A case of obsessive-compulsive neurosis who was listening to the order of his God. Psychiatr Neurol Jpn 84:391–411
33. Berman L (1942) The obsessive compulsive neurosis in children. J Nerv Ment Dis 95:26–39
34. Negishi Y (1976) Obsessive-compulsive neurosis in childhood. Jpn J Clin Psychiatry 5:625–632

Part 5

Psychotic Disorders

Developmental Profiles: Early-Onset Compared to Late-Onset Schizophrenia and Affective Disorders

Yuji Okazaki[1], Kosuke Fujimaru[1], Yoshibumi Nakane[1], Yasutaka Muto[1], Yuji Minami[1], Takahiro Tsujita[1], Jun Uchino[1], Hiromichi Maeda[2], and Tetsuro Fukazawa[3]

Summary. We investigated the developmental profiles of 36 schizophrenics and 14 patients with early-onset (under age 18) affective disorders and compared them to those of 22 schizophrenics and 31 patients with late-onset (35 years old or more but under age 50) affective disorders. These 103 patients were selected, based on age of onset, from 160 schizophrenic and 117 affective patients admitted to Nagasaki University Hospital between 1986 and 1990 who met *Diagnostic and Statistical Manual of Mental Disorders* (*DSM-III or DSM-III-Revised*) criteria. Developmental profiles were delineated by four general factors consisting of nine items that were surveyed in the patients' clinical records: (1) genetic vulnerability (psychiatric illness in first-degree relatives); (2) physical and environmental risk factors (perinatal complications and the loss of either or both parents before age 15); (3) premorbid physical and behavioral problems (delay in motor and speech development, abnormal preferences, physical illness at less than age 18, maladaptation to school, low scholastic achievement); (4) precipitating factors (life events during the year before onset). The patients were classified on the basis of the characteristics of their develop mental profiles. A considerable number in both early-onset groups had genetic vulnerabilities, physical risk factors, and premorbid physical and behavioral problems, although circumstances varied between the groups. Moreover, a considerable number in both late-onset groups had experienced life events during the year before onset that were considered possible precipitating factors. A large number of the late-onset affective disorder patients had genetic vulnerability, whereas a high proportion of the late-onset schizophrenia patients had experienced environmental risk factors. Thus the four groups were fairly well differentiated by their developmental profiles.

Key words. Schizophrenia—Affective disorder—Early-onset—Developmental profile

[1] Department of Neuropsychiatry, Nagasaki University School of Medicine, Sakamoto 1-7-1, Nagasaki City, Nagasaki 852, Japan
[2] Isahaya Mental Hospital, 43-1 Shiromi-cho, Isahaya City, Nagasaki 854, Japan
[3] Department of Psychiatry, Goto-chuo Hospital, 488 Kiba-machi, Fukue City, Nagasaki 853, Japan

Objectives

Schizophrenia that occurs during childhood or adolescence (early-onset schizophrenia) generally manifests severe clinical symptoms and has a poor prognosis. This picture is frequently different from that of schizophrenia that occurs during late adulthood (late-onset schizophrenia). Although possible differences in etiology have not become an issue, some investigators have speculated clinical heterogeneity between them [1, 2]. Early-onset affective disorders are frequently bipolar and show atypical features and rapid cycling. Thus they have been considered to be clinically dissimilar from late-onset affective disorders [3].

Some investigators have regarded brain damage or neurodevelopmental abnormality during the developmental stage from fetus to puberty as the origin of slight brain morphologic abnormalities, such as ventricular enlargement, that are demonstrated by premortem imaging and postmortem study of the brain in some schizophrenics [4–6]. One theory on the etiology of affective disorders, bipolar disorders in particular, proposes disturbances in neurodevelopment [7]. The involvement of genetic factors in the etiology of schizophrenia and affective disorders has been reported in twin and adoption studies The rate of concordance of schizophrenia in monozygotic twins is reported to be as high as 50% [8], whereas that in dizygotic twins is about 15%. These rates are higher than the morbidity risk rate (6.6%) in nontwin siblings [9]. There is an association between the occurrence of schizophrenia in adopted children and the pathologic communication styles of their adopted families [10], suggesting that, in addition to genetic factors, broadly defined environmental factors influence the occurrence or course of the disease. A vulnerability-stress model proposed by Zubin and Spring [11] and the bio-psycho-social model proposed by Ciompi [12] are well known models of the pathogenesis of schizophrenia. With regard to affective disorder, interactions between life events and an individual with a specific vulnerability to an affective disorder are considered important in the multidimensional classification of depression proposed by Kasahara and Kimura [13]. Therefore if schizophrenia and affective disorder have heterogeneous pathogeneses, they may exhibit different longitudinal aspects of development (developmental profiles).

This study was designed to determine the developmental profiles of early-onset schizophrenia and affective disorder compared to those of late-onset schizophrenia and affective disorder by comparing the developmental items for these disorders.

Subjects

The subjects were chosen from 427 patients who were admitted to the psychiatric ward of Nagasaki University Hospital between January 1, 1986, and December 31, 1990. The diagnosis on discharge met the criteria for *Diagnostic and Statistical Manual of Mental Disorders* (*DSM-III* [14] *or DSM-III-Revised* [15]) schizophrenia in 160 patients and for bipolar disorder and major depressive disorder in 117 of the 427 patients. Of these 277 patients, 103 could be assigned to early-onset and late-onset groups. Age at onset was defined as the age when psychotic symptoms (in schizophrenia) or affective symptoms (in bipolar or major depressive disorder) appeared that later resulted in full symptoms that met the diagnostic criteria. According to Nishizono [16] and Kasahara [17], the upper limit of early onset is determined as under 18 years of age. Late onset was defined as onset at 35 years of age or older but

Table 1. Subjects: ages at onset and discharge from hospital.

Group	Schizophrenia			Affective disorder		
	No. of patients[a]	Age at onset	Age at discharge	No. of patients[a]	Age at onset	Age at discharge
Early-onset	36 (15)	15.1 ± 2.0	21.5 ± 6.8	14[b] (9)	14.3 ± 1.2	21.7 ± 6.4
Late-onset	22 (13)	39.2 ± 4.4	47.1 ± 12.0	31[c] (7)	42.3 ± 3.9	48.1 ± 7.1

See text concerning the selection procedure of subjects.
Age at discharge is age at the time of the survey. All results are given as the mean ± standard deviation (years).
There is a significant difference in the distribution of the number of patients with bipolar and depressive disorders between the early-onset and late-onset groups ($\chi^2 = 11.007$, df = 1, $P = 0.0009$) and in the distribution of the number of patients according to sex between the two groups (Fisher's exact probability = 0.0094).
[a] The numbers in parentheses indicate the female subjects in the group.
[b] Includes 11 bipolar and 3 depressive disorder patients.
[c] Includes 8 bipolar and 23 depressive disorder patients.

younger than 50 years. This age range was selected taking into consideration the following facts: The age at onset of schizophrenia was under 50 years in 160 patients; a second peak of affective disorder was observed at ages ranging from 35 to 40 years [18]. Silent cerebral infarctions were frequently detected by magnetic resonance imaging in patients with affective disorder that developed after 50 years of age. Thus because the possibility of heterogeneity may be increased by causal factors [19], the above age range was adopted.

The 103 patients comprised four groups: 36 patients with early-onset schizophrenia (age range 10-17 years, mean ± SD 15.7 ± 2.0 years); 22 with late-onset schizophrenia (35-49 years, 39.2 ± 4.4 years); 14 with early-onset affective disorder (12-16 years, 14.3 ± 1.2 years); and 31 with late-onset affective disorder (36–49 years; 42.3 ± 3.9 years). There was no significant difference in age at discharge between schizophrenia and affective disorder for both early- and late-onset groups (Table 1). The youngest age at onset of affective disorder was 12 years in this survey, which is consistent with the observation by Ishizaka and Takagi [20] that occurrence of depression or manic-depressive illness before age 10 is unlikely. The youngest age at onset of schizophrenia was 10 years, consistent with the observation by Matsumoto [21] that occurrence before age 10 is uncommon when using the criteria for adult schizophrenia. The sex ratio and the frequency of subtypes for early- and late-onset affective disorders were examined. In contrast with the late-onset patients, the proportion of female patients among those with early-onset affective disorder was high, and most of them had bipolar disorder. Thus there were significant differences in the sex ratio and subtype distribution of affective disorder, as shown in Table 1. However, no sex difference has been reported for the onset of manic-depressive psychosis of childhood or adolescence [22]. In female adolescents, cyclic affective disorder has been noted in association with menstruation; however, the bipolar/depressive disorder ratio for early-onset affective patients has not been confirmed. The lifetime morbidity risk for depression in women is believed to be about twice that in men. Depression occurring in relation to reproductive ages (15–45 years) may contribute to the difference [23]. Therefore the sex ratio and subtype distribution in this survey of affective disorder severe enough to require hospitalization may not represent the overall sex ratio or distribu-

Table 2. Items surveyed in the study.

Genetic vulnerability
  Psychiatric illness in first-degree relatives

Physical and environmental risk factors
  Perinatal complications during pregnancy and labor and in the neonate
  Long-term absence or loss of either or both parents before age 15 (excluding absence because of work)

Premorbid physical and behavioral problems
  Distinct delay in motor and speech development compared with standard development
  Abnormal preferences such as those resulting in an unbalanced diet
  Physical illness at less than 18 years of age
  Maladaptation to school accompanied by absence from school occurring at least by 1 year earlier than onset (excluding absence from school within 1 year before onset)
  Low scholastic achievement (achievement rated as 1 or 2 according to 5-grade criteria)

Psychosocial precipitating factors
  Life events out of the individual's control within 1 year before onset.

tion of affective disorder. There was no significant sex difference between early- and late-onset schizophrenia groups.

Methods of Survey

The nine items shown in Table 2 were investigated in 103 patients by admission chart review. When recording the history at admission (including the nine items), the attending and consulting physicians surveyed the patient and family members in detail. When reporting the cases at staff meetings during admission, we carefully discussed omissions in recording. The developmental and life histories recorded in our department were as comprehensive as possible. However, information about childhood was less accurate for some patients in the late-onset group than in the early-onset group because of the parents' death or inadequate recall of information by the patient's siblings. After the records on the corresponding items were transferred to inquiry forms, examiners blindly evaluated whether the records corresponded to the definition of each item. As shown in Table 2, these items were classified into genetic vulnerability, physical and environmental risk factors, premorbid physical and behavioral problems, and psychosocial precipitating factors. Because there was no difference in age at discharge (i.e., the observation period was the same) between the patients with schizophrenia and affective disorder for both the early- and late-onset groups, comparisons of items were possible. Because there were differences in the age of relatives between the early- and late-onset groups, however, strict comparison of family histories of psychiatric disorders was not possible. Intergroup comparison of the history of physical illnesses in the subjects under age 18 was possible because the mean age at discharge was over 20 years even in those with early-onset schizophrenia or affective disorder. For the evaluation of maladaptation to school, cases occurring 1 year before onset were excluded to avoid overlap with the latent onset of a corresponding illness. Life events were defined as significant events that occurred within 1 year before onset but events in which patients voluntarily participated (e.g., leaving a job because of a change of occupation was not adopted, but loss of employment due to bankruptcy was adopted).

Table 3. Comparison of early-onset and late-onset schizophrenia.

Items surveyed	Early-onset group (%)[a] ($n = 36$)	Late-onset group (%)[a] ($n = 22$)	Results of test (significance)
Psychiatric illness in first-degree relatives	27.8	19.0	NS
Perinatal complications	22.9	0	$P < 0.0166$*
Loss of parent(s) before age 15	11.1	31.8	NS
Delay in motor and speech development	13.9	0	NS
Abnormal preferences	8.3	0	NS
Physical illness under age 18	30.6	14.3	NS
Maladaptation to school	22.2	33.3	NS
Low scholastic achievement	30.6	40.0	NS
Life events within 1 year before onset	19.4	42.9	NS

[a] Proportion of patients with a positive item relative to the total number of patients excluding patients for whom there are no data for the item.
* By Fisher's exact probability test; NS, statistically not significant ($P \geq 0.05$).

Results

Comparison of Early-Onset and Late-Onset Schizophrenic Groups

The patients in the early-onset group were younger by at least 20 years on average than those in the late-onset group. Their relatives therefore should also be younger. The frequency of psychiatric illness in first-degree relatives was higher in the early-onset group than in the late-onset group, although the difference was not significant (Table 3). When the difference of at least 20 years was taken into account, the frequency of psychiatric illness in the early-onset group relatives, particularly in siblings and children of probands, was predicted to be even higher in the early-onset group than in the late-onset group. Frequencies of perinatal complications, physical illness under 18 years of age, maladaptation to school, and low scholastic achievement were relatively high in the early-onset group (Table 3). In the late-onset group, by contrast, long-term absence or loss of either or both parents, maladaptation to school, and low scholastic achievement before 15 years of age, and life events within 1 year before the onset in which the patients did not participate were high in frequency (Table 3). There was a significant difference in perinatal complications between the early- and late-onset groups, with a significantly higher frequency in the early-onset group (Table 3).

Comparison of Early-Onset and Late-Onset Affective Disorders

The frequencies of a considerable number of items were high in the early-onset group: In particular, physical illness occurred at less than 18 years of age in at least 50% (Table 4). On the other hand, frequencies of psychiatric illness in first-degree relatives, physical illness at less than 18 years of age, and life events within 1 year before the onset were high in the late-onset group (Table 4). The frequency of psychiatric illness in first-degree relatives was higher in the late-onset group than in the early-onset group, in contrast with the findings for schizophrenia. Because this result may have been influenced by the difference in the period surveyed, which was at least 20

Table 4. Comparison of early-onset and late-onset affective disorders.

Items surveyed	Early-onset group (%)[a] (n = 14)	Late-onset group (%)[a] (n = 31)	Results of test
Psychiatric illness in first-degree relatives	23.1	54.8	NS
Perinatal complications	21.4	0	P < 0.0275*
Loss of parent(s) before age 15	28.6	9.7	NS
Delay in motor and speech development	21.4	0	P > 0.0275*
Abnormal preferences	0	0	NS
Physical illness under age 18	57.1	29.0	NS
Maladaptation to school	30.8	9.7	NS
Low scholastic achievement	35.7	6.5	P > 0.0226*
Life events within 1 year before onset	23.1	61.3	P > 0.0207**

[a] Proportion of patients with a positive item relative to the total number of patients, excluding patients for whom there are no data for item.
* By Fisher's exact probability test; ** by χ^2 test; NS, statistically not significant ($P \geq 0.05$).

years in terms of the mean age of relatives, it is not possible to conclude that the frequency was higher in the late-onset group than in the early-onset group. However, the frequency of life events was significantly higher in the late-onset group (Table 4). Most patients in the late-onset group were men with depressive disorders, suggesting that significant life events are common and were contributing precipitating factors in male patients with depressive disorders. Further comparison revealed significantly higher frequencies of perinatal complications, delay in motor and speech development, and low scholastic achievement in the early-onset group than in the late-onset group (Table 4). The two former items, perinatal complications and delay in motor and speech development, suggest that slight brain organic factors are also involved in the development of early-onset affective disorders. Most of the early-onset affective disorders were bipolar in this survey and were more common in female patients. These findings suggest that early-onset bipolar disorder includes a subgroup in which slight brain organic factors are involved.

Comparison of Early-Onset Schizophrenia and Affective Disorder

The early-onset schizophrenic group was the same as the early-onset affective disorder group in that relatively high frequencies were noted for psychiatric illness in first-degree relatives, perinatal complications, physical illness occurring at less than 18 years of age, maladaptation to school, and low scholastic achievement (Table 5). The two groups were different in that frequencies of long-term absence or loss of either or both parents before 15 years of age, delay in motor and speech development, and life events within 1 year before onset were higher in the early-onset affective disorder (Table 5). Thus there were many items in common in the developmental profiles between the schizophrenic and affective groups. However, when the contents of the items were investigated, they were not necessarily similar.

Psychiatric illness in first-degree relatives was determined not by directly interviewing all family members but, rather, from information provided by key persons during treatment of the proband. Therefore it is not an exact indicator: The frequency of the disorder tends to be reported as lower than the actual frequency, and the

Table 5. Comparison of early-onset affective disorder and schizophrenia.

Items surveyed	Affective disorder (%)[a] (n = 14)	Schizophrenia (%)[a] (n = 36)
Psychiatric illness in first-degree relatives	23.1	27.8
Perinatal complications	21.4	22.9
Loss of parent(s) before age 15	28.6	11.1
Delay in motor and speech development	21.4	13.9
Abnormal preferences	0	8.3
Physical illness under age 18	57.1	30.6
Maladaptation to school	30.8	22.2
Low scholastic achievement	35.7	30.6
Life events within 1 year before onset	23.1	19.4

None of the results of the tests were statistically significant ($P \geq 0.05$).
[a] Proportion of patients with a positive item relative to the total number of patients, excluding patients for whom there were no data for the item.

disorder itself may not be correctly identified. Some relatives of patients with early-onset schizophrenia had been reported or diagnosed variously as a visit to a psychiatric clinic, tics, alcoholism, depression, manic-depressive psychosis, borderline state with suicidal attempt, reactive psychosis, paranoid schizophrenia, schizophrenia, and disorganized schizophrenia. Schizophrenia was the highest in frequency, but alcohol-related disorders and affective disorders were also frequently reported. These data suggested that not only schizophrenia but also alcoholism and affective disorders were reported among the relatives of the probands with early-onset schizophrenia. As noted by Gottesman and Shields [8], a high frequency of alcoholism was suggested by Rüdin of the Munich school to be seen among the relatives of schizophrenics. The results of the present survey tended to be consistent with this finding. On the other hand, neurosis, school refusal, depression, manic-depressive psychosis, experience of possession, schizophrenia, and epilepsy also were reported among first-degree relatives of the probands with early-onset affective disorders. However, because most of the relatives had depression or bipolar disorder and the other diagnoses were observed in one relative each, the frequencies of illnesses more closely related to the disorder of the probands were considered higher in first-degree relatives of patients with early-onset affective disorder than in those with early-onset schizophrenia.

The perinatal complications in the early-onset schizophrenic group were relatively serious, consisting of asphyxia, blepharoptosis due to vacuum extraction, cord entanglement, preterm labor, and preterm amniorrehexis. The perinatal complications in the early-onset affective disorder group were preterm labor resulting in a premature infant and cyanosis due to vacuum extraction. These problems were generally milder than in the early-onset schizophrenia group.

The main physical illnesses under 18 years of age in the early-onset schizophrenic group were infectious and allergic diseases, such as persistently high fever, otitis media, cold-induced dehydration, pneumonia, infantile asthma, atopic dermatitis, itching, pyelonephritis, nephritis, hypotension, and tics. The physical illnesses under 18 years of age in the early-onset affective disorder group were frequently febrile convulsion between 2 and 6 years of age, afebrile convulsion during childhood, fever of unknown origin, goiter, hepatic dysfunction, hepatitis antigen carrier, appendicitis, and spondylosis. Illnesses such as convulsive disorders, which differed from the

Table 6. Comparison of late-onset affective disorder and schizophrenia.

Items surveyed	Affective disorder (%)[a] (n = 31)	Schizophrenia (%)[a] (n = 22)	Results of test
Psychiatric illness in first-degree relatives	54.8	19.0	P < 0.0099**
Perinatal complications	0	0	NS
Loss of parent(s) before age 15	9.7	31.8	P < 0.0478*
Delay in motor and speech development	0	0	NS
Abnormal preferences	0	0	NS
Physical illness under age 18	29.0	14.3	NS
Maladaptation to school	9.7	33.3	P < 0.0485*
Low scholastic achievement	6.5	40.0	P < 0.005**
Life events within 1 year before onset	61.3	42.9	NS

[a] Proportion of patients with a positive item relative to the total number of patients, excluding patients for whom there were no data for the item.
* By Fisher's exact probability test; ** by χ^2 test; NS, statistically not significant ($P \geq 0.05$).

physical illnesses seen in the early-onset schizophrenic group, were observed in the early-onset affective disorder group.

Thus early-onset schizophrenia and affective disorder showed similar profiles of developmental items, but these items differed in content.

Comparison of Late-Onset Schizophrenia and Affective Disorder

The late-onset schizophrenia and affective disorder groups showed different developmental profiles. The frequencies of environmental risk factors such as long-term absence and loss of either or both parents before 15 years of age were significantly higher in the schizophrenia group than in the affective disorder group; furthermore, the schizophrenia patients showed maladaptation to school and low scholastic achievement (Table 6), indicating premorbid low functioning. On the other hand, the frequency of psychiatric illness in first-degree relatives was significantly higher in the affective disorder group than in the schizophrenia group. The frequencies of significant life events within 1 year before onset were high in both groups: at least 60% in the affective disorder group and nearly 43% in the schizophrenia group. The frequency of psychiatric illnesses in first-degree relatives of late-onset affective disorder patients was high (Table 6) and widely distributed: a visit to a psychiatric clinic, suicide, alcohol dependence, insomnia, neurosis, depression, postpartum depression, puerperal psychosis, manic-depressive psychosis, hypomania, neurasthenia, paranoid schizophrenia, schizophrenia, and senile dementia. In contrast, the frequency of psychiatric illness in first-degree relatives of late-onset schizophrenia group was low; and a history of psychiatric admission, suicide because of neurosis, mild depression, manic-depressive psychosis, alcoholism, or paranoid schizophrenia was reported. That is, only one relative was reported as having schizophrenia.

Thus among the relatives of the patients with late-onset groups, psychiatric illnesses in the relatives were less closely related to those in the probands than in early-onset groups, particularly in the schizophrenia group. The frequencies of illnesses in first-degree relatives closely related to those of the probands were highest for the late-onset affective disorder, followed by early-onset schizophrenia, then late-onset affective disorder, and finally late-onset schizophrenia.

Some schizophrenic patients experienced long-term absence or loss of either or both parents before 15 years of age: separation from the mother (a mistress) when 6 months old, adoption immediately after birth, being sent to a geisha house when 13 years old; parent's divorce when 1 year old; father's death in battle; and mother's death from disease when 10 years old. Only three patients with affective disorder experienced significant life events; all three experienced parent death at less than 5 years of age. Thus the schizophrenia group included more severe cases of separation from parents than did those in the affective disorder group, which seemed to depend on the family's situation.

The physical illnesses that occurred at less than 18 years of age in the patients with affective disorders were febrile convulsion, asthma, sinusitis, appendicitis, malaria-like pyrexia, paratyphoid fever, pleuritis, tuberculosis, ovariotomy at school age, and gastric ulcer; thus various infectious diseases were observed as well as febrile convulsion. The schizophrenic group showed the same type of illnesses as the early-onset schizophrenic group (pneumonia, high fever, and asthma), although the number of cases was much lower. The types of physical illnesses under 18 years of age in the late-onset groups were different in the schizophrenia group from those seen in the affective disorder group despite the fact that these patients had lived during same 18-year period.

The life events frequently observed in late-onset affective disorder group were personnel reorganization at work, transfer to a new location soon after purchasing a home, promotion, moving into a new house, signs of physical disease, athletic bone fracture, child's failure to pass an entrance examination, child's illness and inducement of parents to join a new religion, child's suicide, parent's illness or worsening of symptoms or hospitalization, relative's hospitalization or divorce or death, and disaster-related debt. These events were characterized by change in occupational status, occupational transfer, promotion to a higher occupational position, changes in residence, injury and illness, negative affairs of family members, and so on. The life events frequently observed in the late-onset schizophrenia group included building a new house not with the patient's approval, business trip, personnel reorganization at work, tuberculosis, parent's illness or death, disclosure of adultery, family's opposition to marriage, or husband's political candidacy. Building a new house, personnel reorganization, and family member's illness or death were common items in both groups, but the frequency of occupational problems was much higher in the affective disorder group than in the schizophrenia group. General conclusions should be cautiously drawn because the adaptation to life before onset may have already been poor in the schizophrenic group, but it is clear that the life events that the two groups encountered 1 year before onset may have been considerably different.

When components of the corresponding items were investigated in the late-onset groups, however, some items showed less distinct differences than those observed between the early-onset groups. "Evaluation of the item psychiatric illnesses in first-degree relatives," in particular, revealed results that may have been due to the inhomogeneity of the late-onset groups. Late-onset disorders may develop through interactions with environmental risk factors (particularly in the schizophrenia group) or life events (particularly in the affective disorder group). Regardless of the reason, the developmental profiles of the late-onset groups were different from those of the early-onset groups.

Table 7. Summary of study.

Factor	Affective disorder (%)		Schizophrenia (%)	
	Early onset	Late onset	Early onset	Late onset
Genetic vulnerability	20+	50+	20+	
Risk factors				
Physical	20+[a]		20+[a]	
Environmental	20+			20+[b]
Premorbid manifestations of pathology				
Physical	50+[a]	20+	20+	
Behavioral	20+[a]		20+	20+[b]
Psychosocial precipitating factors	20+	50+[a]		20+

The results are the observed percent of patients with the factor in the particular subject group.
[a] Significantly more frequent than in any group of the same disease whose age at onset is different.
[b] Significantly more frequent than in another disease group whose age at onset is the same.

Discussion

Table 7 summarizes the items that were relatively frequently (at least 20%) and frequently (at least 50%) observed and that showed significant intergroup differences. In the affective disorders group the frequencies of genetic vulnerability (psychiatric illness in first-degree relatives) and psychosocial precipitating factors (life events within 1 year before onset) were high regardless of age at onset, whereas the frequency of psychosocial risk factors was significantly higher in the late-onset group. In the early-onset group the frequencies of genetic vulnerability, precipitating factors, physical and environmental risk factors (perinatal complications, long-term absence or loss of either or both parents before age 15), and premorbid physical and behavioral problems (delay in motor and speech development, physical illness at less than 18 years of age, maladaptation to school, low scholastic achievement) were high; the frequency of physical illness at less than age 18 was particularly high. Physical and environmental risk factors in addition to genetic vulnerability are thought to be involved in the pathogenesis of early-onset affective disorders, resulting in the manifestation of disadvantages in neural, physical, and intellectual functions and adaptive behaviors. Such characteristics were suggested in the early-onset affective disorder, which showed a different profile from the late-onset group that was closely related to psychosocial risk factors.

The developmental profile of the early-onset schizophrenia group was different from that of the late-onset schizophrenia group. The frequencies of environmental risk factors (long-term absence or loss of either or both parents before age 15) and psychosocial precipitating factors (life events 1 year before onset) were high in the late-onset group, whereas the frequencies of physical risk factors (perinatal complications), genetic vulnerability, and premorbid manifestation of physical pathology (physical illness at less than 18 years of age) were high in the early-onset group. The frequency of premorbid manifestations of behavioral problems (maladaptation to school, low scholastic achievement) was high in both early-onset and late-onset schizophrenia groups.

The common finding observed in the late-onset affective disorder group and the late-onset schizophrenic group was a high frequency of psychosocial precipitating factors. There were marked differences in other items; the frequencies of genetic vulnerability and premorbid manifestation of physical pathology (physical illness at less than 18 years of age) were high in the affective disorder group, whereas those for environmental risk factors and premorbid manifestation of behavioral problems (premorbid maladaptation to school and low scholastic achievement) were high in the late-onset schizophrenia group.

In early-onset affective disorder and early-onset schizophrenia, the frequencies of genetic vulnerability, physical risk factors (perinatal complications), and premorbid manifestations of physical and behavioral problems were high, and there were a number of items with relatively high frequency common between the two groups. These pathogenetic factors and premorbid manifestations of physical and behavioral problems in the early-onset affective disorder and schizophrenia are considered consistent with such previous findings as neurodevelopmental abnormalities, suggested by minor physical anomalies, and brain morphological abnormalities seen by premortem in vivo imaging and postmortem study [2, 7]. This finding may explain in part the general finding that the prognosis of early-onset schizophrenia is poor in many cases. Early-onset affective disorders are likely to follow the course of bipolar disorders, which, as discussed by Kasahara and Kimura [13], may indicate the premorbid presence of a physical base in which bipolar disorders show more marked lowering of mental energy level than is seen with depressive disorder. Thus stratification of schizophrenic and affective patients by age at onset suggests that the assessment of psychopathology based on life cycle, developed in psychology and clinical psychopathology [16, 17], can provide fruitful results for the biological study of the pathogenesis of mental disorders.

Because the present survey was done retrospectively, it was subject to various limitations, particularly the lack of a common evaluation using a structured interview or a rating scale. Therefore the reproducibility of the findings concerning developmental profiles, which were thought to be different owing to age at onset and diseases in this survey, should be demonstrated by careful and prospective investigation.

Acknowledgment. This study was performed as part the Studies of the Project Team on the Pathogenesis and Psychopathology of Behavioral and Emotional Disorders in Childhood and Adolescence, supported by a grant from the National Center of Neurology and Psychiatry (NCNP) of the Ministry of Health and Welfare, Japan, in 1991.

References

1. Sasaki T, Okazaki Y (1991) Age at onset in the diagnosis and symptomatology of schizophrenia (in Japanese). Arch Psychiatr Diagn Clin Eval 2:279–289
2. Castle DJ, Murray RM (1991) The neurodevelopmental basis of sex differences in schizophrenia [editorial]. Psychol Med 21:565–575
3. Kunugi H, Hirose T (1991) Diagnostic and therapeutic issues in terms of the age at onset in mood disorders (in Japanese). Arch Psychiatr Diagn Clin Eval 2:291–304
4. Murray RM (1987) Is schizophrenia a neurodevelopmental disorder? BMJ 295:681–682
5. Crow TJ, Ball J, Bloom SR, et al (1989) Schizophrenia as an anomaly of development of cerebral asymmetry. Arch Gen Psychiatry 46:1145–1150
6. Okazaki Y (1992) A selected review of neurodevelopmental theories of schizophrenia (in Japanese). Jpn J Clin Psychiatry 21:205–218

7. Nasrallah HA (1991) Neurodevelopmental aspects of bipolar affective disorder [editoral]. Biol Psychiatry 29:1–2
8. Gottesman II, Shields J (1982) Schizophrenia: an epigenetic puzzle. Cambridge University Press, Cambridge, pp 101–113
9. Inouye E (1975) Clinical genetics. In: Kaketa K , Okuma T, Shimazono Y, Takahashi R (eds) Current encyclopedia of psychiatry IIC (in Japanese). Nakayama Shoten, Tokyo, pp 59–117
10. Tienari P, Sorri A, Lahti I, et al (1987) Genetic and psychosocial factors in schizophrenia. Schizophr Bull 13:477–484
11. Zubin J, Spring B (1977) Vulnerability—a new view of schizophrenia. J Abnorm Psychol 86:103–126
12. Ciompi L (1989) The dynamics of complex biological-psychosocial systems: four fundamental psycho-biological mediators in the long-term evolution of schizophrenia. Br J Psychiatry 155(suppl 5):15–21
13. Kasahara Y, Kimura B (1975) For a classification of depressive states (in Japanese). Psychiatr Neurol Jpn 77:715–735
14. American Psychiatric Association (1980) Diagnostic and statistical manual of mental disorders 3rd ed (DSM-III). American Psychiatric Association, Washington, DC
15. American Psychiatric Association (1987) Diagnostic and statistical manual of mental disorders, 3rd ed-revised (DSM-III-R). American Psychiatric Association, Washington, DC
16. Nishizono M (1988) A proposal of life cycle psychiatry. In: Nishizono M (ed) Life cycle psychiatry (in Japanese). Igaku-Shoin, Tokyo, pp 1–17
17. Kasahara Y (1976) Current psychopathology in adolescents. In: Kasahara Y, Shimizu M, Ito K (eds) Psychopathology of adolescents. Kobundo, Tokyo, pp 3–27
18. Nakane Y, Okazaki Y, Uchino J, et al (1992) Study on neuropsychological and developmental factors related to the pathogenesis of childhood/adolescent onset schizophrenia and affective disorder. In: Wakabayashi S (chief): Annual report of the project team of studies on the pathogenesis and psychopathology of behavioral and emotional disorders in childhood and adolescence in 1991 (in Japanese), pp 99–104
19. Okazaki Y, Nakane Y (1990) Senile depression: the significance of subcortical lacunar infarcts (in Japanese). Aging Dis 44:1318–1325
20. Ishizaka Y, Takagi R (1987) Depressive states in children (in Japanese). Jpn J Clin Psychiatry 16:701–708
21. Matsumoto H (1990) Childhood and adolescent psychiatric disorders: current topics. I. Schizophrenia (in Japanese). Seishinka Chiryogaku 5:1389–1397
22. Kaku R, Hanada M (1991) Sex differences in child and adolescent psychiatric disorders (in Japanese). Arch Psychiatr Diagn Clin Eval 2:99–111
23. Whilhelm K, Parker G (1989) Is sex necessarily a risk factor to depression? Psychol Med 19:401–413

Clinical Study of Childhood Schizophrenia

Hideo Matsumoto

Summary. Nineteen schizophrenic children who met the diagnostic criteria of DSM-III were investigated. They were less than 15 years old at the onset of their disease. Comparing the clinical features and Rorschach test results of the childhood schizophrenia group (group C) with those of the adult schizophrenia group (group A), the following characteristics of child schizophrenia were noted. In terms of clinical features: (1) More first-born patients were observed. (2) More prodromal symptoms and latent-onset types were found. (3) Some of the patients had visual hallucinations. (4) The contents of the auditory hallucinations were less clearly described, and the duration was more transitional. (5) Few patients had systematized delusions. (6) Labile mood was commonly observed. (7) Most of the patients had obsessive compulsive symptoms/signs. The Rorschach test results showed a lower value in deviant verbalization, and more real descriptions were found. The results correlated with the clinical symptoms/signs. I then classified the patients with childhood schizophrenia according to the main clinical symptoms/signs after the onset of schizophrenia. They comprised two groups: the flat (F) group and the unstable (U) group. The main clinical symptoms of group F were gradual changes in character, abulia, and autism. In contrast, those of group U were hallucination and delusions. According to the Rorschach test results, the patients of group F had poor psychic energies and flat emotions. In contrast, the patients of group U did not have debilitated psychic energies, lessened volition, or decreased mental acuity. They did have a poor ability to understand reality and poor control of affect. These Rorschach results confirm the clinical features of groups F and U.

Key words. Schizoprenia—Childhood—Rorschach test

Introduction

Schizophrenia during childhood has long been discussed, but its definition has been unclear. The lower age limit at the onset of schizophrenia is a matter of discussion. Furthermore schizophrenia and infantile autism have often been confused. From the late 1960s to the 1970s, Rutter and colleagues [1, 2] and Kolvin and Ounsted [3]

Department of Psychiatry, National Sanatorium Tenryu Hospital, 4201-2 Oro, Hamakita City, Shizuoka 434, Japan reported that infantile autism was associated mainly with verbal and cognitive impairments and was fundamentally different from schizophrenia. The *Diagnostic and Statistical Manual of Mental Disorders* (DSM-III) [4] in 1980 classified infantile autism as a developmental disorder, so it was clearly distinguished from schizophrenia.

Because of the confused history of childhood schizophrenia and infantile autism, few studies on childhood schizophrenia based on any defined criteria have been reported. This chapter describes an investigation of childhood schizophrenia in terms of the following points: (1) diagnosis of patients according to the DSM-III criteria; (2) examination of characteristics of childhood schizophrenia compared with those of adult schizophrenia; (3) classification of childhood schizophrenia into clinical subgroups; and (4) analysis of Rorschach test data.

Subjects and Methods

Subjects

The subjects consisted of 19 schizophrenic children (8 boys, 11 girls) who had been treated at the Department of Psychiatry, Hamamatsu University School of medicine from April 1980 to March 1986. All the subjects met the DSM-III diagnostic criteria when they were less than 15 years of age. The ages of the patients at the onset of schizophrenia ranged from 9 years 7 months to 15 years 11 months. Their ages at presentation ranged from 9 years 7 months to 16 years 8 months (average 14 years 2 months).

Clinical Assessment

The subjects were examined clinically as follows: clinical symptoms/signs, age at onset, medical treatment from onset to presentation, genetic factors, premorbid personality, personal history, type of onset, electroencephalography (EEG), computed tomography (CT) scan of the head, and treatment.

Comparison with Adult Schizophrenia

Twenty patients with schizophrenia were selected at random among patients more than 18 years of age who were diagnosed as having schizophrenia according to the DSM-III criteria at our institution. The ages of the patients at the onset of adult schizophrenia ranged from 18 to 26 years (average 22 years 11 months). Clinical symptoms/signs of childhood schizophrenia were compared with those of adult schizophrenia.

Classification According to Main Clinical Symptoms/Signs

Classification of childhood schizophrenia into subgroups was attempted based on the main clinical symptoms/signs that appeared after the onset of childhood schizophrenia. The subjects were classified into two groups: a flat (F) group and an unstable (U) group. The main clinical symptoms/signs of group F were gradual changes in character, abulia, and autism; those of group U were hallucinations and delusions.

Analysis of Rorschach Test Data

The Rorschach test was performed on patients with either childhood schizophrenia or adult schizophrenia within about 1 year after the onset of their disease, when their psychiatric conditions were relatively stable. As a control group, 10 normal children (five boys, five girls) were subjected to the Rorschach test. The ages of the patients with childhood schizophrenia when undergoing Rorschach testing ranged from 10 years 6 months to 16 years 8 months (average 14 years 4 months). The ages of the patients with adult schizophrenia ranged from 19 years to 27 years 7 months (average 24 years). The ages of the normal children ranged from 13 years to 15 years 4 months (average 14 years 5 months).

The analyses were as follows: (1) comparison between the childhood schizophrenia group (group C) and the adult schizophrenia group (group A) by Rorschach test; and (2) comparison among group F, group U, and group C by Rorschach test.

Results

Clinical Features of Childhood Schizophrenia

Tables 1, 2, and 3 show the backgrounds and clinical features of the patients with childhood schizophrenia.

Clinical Symptoms/Signs

Only one patient (case 1) had catatonic symptoms/signs (e.g., excitement, stupor, echolalia, waxy flexibility, coprolalia, and mannerisms). Most of the patients presented with abnormalities in actions and words. The main symptoms were abnormal behavior ($n = 11$, 57.9%), monologue ($n = 8$, 42.1%); inappropriate smiling ($n = 8$, 42.1%), and obsessive compulsive behavior ($n = 4$, 21.1%). The abnormal behaviors included wandering impulsive action, and violence.

Only four patients (21.1%) had had a flattened affect since the onset. Six patients (31.6%) showed oversensitivity and instability in their interpersonal relationships and a labile mood. Although auditory hallucinations were found in 16 patients (84.2%), few patients could describe the details clearly. Three patients (15.8%) complained of visual hallucinations. None of the patients had had a systematized delusion, although six (31.6%) had delusions of persecution and three (15.8%) had delusions of being possessed.

Age at Onset

Only the patient (no. 1) presented with symptoms of schizophrenia at less than 10 years of age; all the other patients had symptoms when they were older than 10 years. The ages of some patients at the onset of their schizophrenia could not be clearly defined.

Medical Treatment from Onset

The patients whose ages at onset were specified came to our hospital about 10 months after the onset of schizophrenia.

Table 1. Childhood schizophrenia patients: general characteristics.

Pt. no.	Sex	Age at onset (y:m)	Age (at presentation)	Family organization	Genetic factors	Premorbid personality
1	M	9:7	9:7	F, M, GM, YB, YS	−	Oversensitive, introverted, unsociable
2	M	13:4	13:4	F, M	−	Oversensitive, timid, selfish
3	M	~14:0	14:7	F, M, EB	−	Oversensitive, introverted, nervous
4	M	14:0	14:3	F, M, EB, YB, YS	−	Extroverted, not fussy
5	M	14:3	14:3	F, M, YB, YS	−	Bright, oversensitive
6	M	14:6	14:6	F, M, EB, YB,	+	Nervous, selfish, silent, strong sense of responsibility
7	M	~15:0	15:0	F, M, YB	+	Introverted, selfish, nervous, obstinate
8	M	15:0	15:1	F, M, YS	−	Introverted, meek
9	F	11:10	12:0	F, M, GF, GM, YB	+	Introverted, obstinate, meticulous
10	F	13:0	13:0	F, M, GM, YS	+	Selfish, dependent, nervous, meticulous
11	F	13:4	13:4	F, M, GM	+	Oversensitive, meek, unsociable
12	F	13:6	13:6	F, M, ES	−	Oversensitive, introverted, timid
13	F	13:7	14:2	F, M, YS	−	Oversensitive, selfish
14	F	~14:0	14:8	F, M, GM, YS	−	Introverted, nervous, unsociable
15	F	14:0	14:6	F, M, YB	+	Competitive, bright
16	F	14:6	15:0	F, M, YB	−	Introverted, meek, silent
17	F	14:11	15:5	F, M, YB	+	Timid, nervous, oversensitive
18	F	15:10	16:8	M, YS	−	Introverted, oversensitive, rigid, dependent
19	F	15:11	16:3	F, YB	−	Nervous, meek, dependent

F, father; M, mother; GM, grandmother; YB, younger brother; YS, younger sister; EB, elder brother; GF, grandfather; ES, elder sister; y:m, years:months.

Family Organization

Two patients (nos. 18, 19) had a single parent because of divorce. Among the 19 young schizophrenics, 14 patients (73.7%) were first-born.

Genetic Factors

Seven patients (36.8%) had relatives within third-degree limits who had a psychotic disorder.

Premorbid Personality

Although most of the patients had a premorbid personality (e.g., introversion, oversensitivity, unsociability, nervousness), patients 4, 6, and 15 had an extroverted premorbid personality and many friends.

Table 2. Childhood schizophrenia patients: personal history.

Pt. no.	Abnormalities at birth	Early childhood	First period of opposition	During early childhood	Adaptation	
					During childhood	School performance
1	Forceps delivery	Cyclic vomiting	–	Plays alone, strange behaviors since age 6 years	Hyperkinetic, isolated, strange behaviors	Average
2	Neonatal asphyxia	Strabismus	+	Selfish, obstinate, and disobedient	Active, has few friends	Good
3	Breech presentation		–	Plays alone	Has few friends, a bullied child	Good
4			–	Active	Active, a leading figure	Good
5			–	Hyperkinetic	Strange person	Poor
6		Bronchial asthma	?	Bright and has many friends	Has many friends, bright	Average
7		Head injury by traffic accident (at age 2 years)	–	Depressed	Honor student	Good
8			–	Obedient and meek	Earnest	Average
9			–	Dull, isolated	Isolated	Average
10			+	Plays with everyone	Has few friends isolated	Average
11			–	Plays alone	Has few friends	Good
12			–	Obedient, anxious	Has few friends	Poor
13			–	Meek, plays alone	Obedient	Average
14			+	Plays alone	Has few friends	Average
15	Forceps delivery		+	Meek	Has many friends	Average
16	Congenital dislocation of hip, cephalhematoma	Head injury and unconsciousness (at age 2 years)	+	Obedient	Obedient, meek	Average
17	Cephalhematoma	Strabismus	–	Meek, plays alone	Isolated	Average
18	Breech presentation, neonatal asphyxia	Head injury (at age 3 years)	–	Obedient	Isolated	Average
19			?	Plays alone		Average

Table 3. Symptoms exhibited by schizophrenic children in study.

Pt. no.	Prodromal symptoms		Main symptoms	Other symptoms					Type of onset	Group
	Symptoms	Onset		Abnormal behaviors	Abnormal moods	Thought disorders	Hallucinations	Delusions		
1	Hyperkinetic, strange behavior and speech	4y	Incoherence	excitement, stupor, echolalia, waxy flexibility, coprolalia		Incoherence	Aud (content not clear); visual	Delusional mood (transitional)	Latent	
2	Schoold refusal, depers	3y	Aud hall, depers	Monologue, inapp smile autism, violence		Depers, obs-comp ideas	Aud (content not clear)		Latent	U
3	Anxiety, phobia, sleep disturbance, violence	3y	Character changes, abulia, autism	Obs-comp behaviors, abulia, autism	Blunted feeling	Depers		Persecution (transitional)	Latent	F
4	Overwork, appetite loss, few words	2m	Delusions of reference and guilt	Obs-comp behaviors, impulsive action		Obs-comp ideas	Aud (content not clear,transitional)	Reference and guilt	Acute	U
5			Aud hall			Easily influenced, broadcast thoughts	Aud		Acute	U
6	School refusal, hypobulia	7m	Aud hall, monologue	Wandering, monologue, inapp smile, autism	Labile mood	Easily influenced, thought deprivation	Aud (thought resonance)	Possession, reference	S.acute	U
7	School refusal, hypobulia, lying	4y	Abulia, autism	Monologue, inapp smile, abulia, autism					Latent	F
8	School refusal, hypobulia	4m	Abulia	Monologue, impulsive action, violence			Aud (content not clear); visual		S.acute	F
9	Monologue	1y	Aud hall, persecution delusions	Obs-comp behaviors, monologue, inapp smile	Labile mood	Obs-comp ideas, depers	Aud (persecution, thought resonance)	Persecution, observation	S.acute	U
10			Aud hall, possession delusions	Violence, impulsive action		Easily influenced, thought insertion	Aud	Possession	Acute	U
11	Attention disorder	1m	Aud hall, possession delusions	Excitement, stupor, impulsive action	Labile mood	Broadcast thoughts, easily influenced	Aud (persecution, reference)	Possession, persecution, reference	Acute	

Table 3. *Continued.*

Pt. no.	Prodromal symptoms		Main symptoms	Other symptoms					Type of onset	Group
	Symptoms	Onset		Abnormal behaviors	Abnormal moods	Thought disorders	Hallucinations	Delusions		
12	School refusal, anxiety, attention disorder	2 y	Abulia, autism	Strange behavior and speech, monologue, inapp smile	Blunted feeling	Blocked thoughts	Aud (content not clear)	Persecution (transitional)	Latent	F
13			Abulia, autism	Violence, strange behavior and speech, inapp smile			Aud (content not clear, transitional)		S.acute	F
14	Depressed mood, impulsive action	3 y	Delusional mood, labile mood	Wandering, excitement, impulsive action	Labile mood	Depers	Aud (content not clear, transitional)	Delusional mood	Latent	U
15	Strange behavior and speech	2 y	Abulia	Tic, coprolalia, monologue	Blunted feeling		Aud (content not clear, transitional)		Latent	F
16	Appetite loss	1 y	Abulia, autism	Impulsive action, inapp smile,	Blunted feeling	Broadcast thoughts	Aud (content not clear)	Persecution	S.acute	F
17			Autism, depers	Abulia	Labile mood	Depers		Delusional mood	Acute	F
18	School refusal, obs-comp behavior	4 m	Autism	Obs-comp behaviors, runs away from home		Gender identity disorder	Aud (persecution)		Latent	F
19			Aud hall, persecution delusions	Excitement	Labile mood		Aud (content not clear); visual	Persecution	Acute	U

aud, auditory; obs-comp, obsessive compulsive; S.acute, subacute; hall, hallucination; depers, depersonalization; inapp, inappropriate; U, unstable; F, flat; y, years; m, months.

Personal History

Only five patients (26.3%) demonstrated the first period of opposition during early childhood. Most patients, with the exception of patients 9 and 12, had grades above average in elementary school. All 11 female patients had experienced menarche before the onset of schizophrenia.

Types of Onset

The onset of schizophrenia was classified into three types: acute, subacute, and latent. The patients with acute onset ($n = 6$, 31.6%) had only a brief prodromal phase, those of subacute onset ($nM = 5$, 26.3%) had a prodromal period of several months to 10 months, and those of latent onset ($n = 8$, 42.1%) had a prodromal period of several years.

Prodromal Symptoms

Fourteen patients (73.7%) had prodromal symptoms. Six patients (nos. 2, 6, 7, 8, 12, 18) exhibited school refusal and hypobulia, and five patients (nos. 1, 3, 4, 14, 15) had abnormal behaviors, such as using made-up words, and exhibiting strange behaviors, impulsive behaviors, and violence.

Electroencephalography and Computed Tomography of the Head

Abnormal EEG results were found in six patients (nos. 2, 8, 9, 11, 14, 16): patient 2, diffusely mixed θ waves (5–7 cycles per second, or cps); patient 8, a tendency toward diffuse α waves; patient 9, 6 cps positive waves in the left temporal area; patient 11, a tendency toward diffuse α waves and a build-up of, and poor recovery from, hyperventilation; patient 14, slow α waves of 8 cps; and patient 16, 6 cps positive waves in the right occipital area and diffusely mixed θ waves of 5–7 cps.

Treatment

Sixteen of the patients (84.2%) required hospitalization (Table 4). Table 4 shows the daily administered dose of major tranquilizers during April 1986.

Adult Schizophrenia

Clinical Features

Table 5 shows the clinical features of the adults in our study with schizophrenia. Of these patients, 10 had hebephrenic schizophrenia (six men, four women) and 10 had the paranoid type (five men, five women). In eight cases the patients were first-born (40%), in nine cases they were second-born (45%), and in three cases they were third-born (15%). Eight patients (50%) had a genetic factor (in four cases it was not known). The patients (50%) had prodromal symptoms, which were mainly hypobulia ($n = 7$). The types of onset were acute ($n = 12$, 60%) subacute ($n = 4$, 20%), or latent ($n = 4$, 20%). The clinical symptoms observed were violence and wandering ($M = 11$, 55%), monologue ($n = 8$, 40%), inappropriate smiling ($n = 8$, 40%), obsessive compulsive behavior ($n = 1$, 5%), and auditory hallucination ($n = 14$, 70%). None of the patients complained of visual hallucinations. Ten patients were able to describe the details of their auditory hallucinations clearly. Sixteen patients (80%) had some delusion that

Table 4. Treatment of child schizophrenics.

Pt. no.	Hospitalization	Daily administered dose	EEG
1	+	Chlorpromazine 450 mg, levomepromazine 75 mg, carbamazepine 600 mg	Normal
2	+	Chlorpromazine 75 mg, thioridazine 30 mg	Abnormal
3	−	Chlorpromazine 85 mg, timiperone 3 mg	Normal
4	+	Levomepromazine 125 mg, timiperone 24 mg	Normal
5	−	Haloperidol 3 mg, thioridazine 40 mg	Normal
6	+	Chlorpromazine 200 mg, haloperidol 6 mg	Normal
7	+	Carpipramine 200 mg, levomepromazine 15 mg	Normal
8	−	Perphenazine 6 mg, thioridazine 30 mg	Abnormal
9	+	Chlorpromazine 45 mg, haloperidol 4.5 mg, levomepromazine 40 mg	Abnormal
10	+	Haloperidol 4.75 mg, thioridazine 60 mg, levomepromazine 20 mg	Normal
11	+	Haloperidol 4.5 mg, propericiazine 75 mg, levomepromazine 40 mg	Abnormal
12	+	Chlorpromazine 400 mg, haloperidol 12 mg, levomepromazine 120 mg	Normal
13	+	Chlorpromazine 250 mg, perphenazine 12 mg, haloperidol 11 mg	Normal
14	+	Chlorpromazine 250 mg, haloperidol 9 mg	Abnormal
15	+	Haloperidol 2.25 mg, propericiazine 100 mg	Normal
16	+	Chlorpromazine 250 mg, timiperone 12 mg	Abnormal
17	+	Chlorpromazine 150 mg, haloperidol 6 mg	Normal
18	+		Normal
19	+	Perphenazine 30 mg	Normal

was mostly of persecution and reference. Three patients has systematized delusions, and none showed catatonic symptoms/signs.

Clinical Features: Childhood Versus Adult Schizophrenia

Compared to the patients with adult schizophrenia (group A), the following characteristics are observed in the patients with childhood schizophrenia (group C). More first-born patients were observed. There were no differences between the two groups regarding the presence of a genetic factor. Prodromal symptoms, latent-onset type, obsessive compulsive symptoms, and labile mood were observed more often in the children. The contents of the auditory hallucinations were less clearly described, and their duration was more transitional. Visual hallucinations were reported only by children, whereas systematized delusions were found only in the adults.

Classification of Childhood Schizophrenia

Nine patients (three boys, six girls) were classified into group F and eight patients (four boys, four girls) into group U. The clinical features of each group are as follows:

1. *Clinical symptoms*: Though hallucination and delusion were observed in group F, they were transitional or not severe. The most frequently observed symptom/sign was gradual changes in character in group F. In contrast, the main symptoms/signs of

Table 5. Adult Schizophrenics: general characteristics.

Pt. no.	Sex	Age at onset[a]	Birth order/ siblings	Genetic factor	Prodromal symptoms		Main symptoms					Type of onset
					Symptom	Onset	Abnormal behaviors	Abnormal moods	Thought disorders	Hallucinations	Delusions	
Hebephrenic schizophrenia												
1	M	18:1	2/2	+	High school dropout, hypobulia, violence	6 m	Violence, abulia, autism		Incoherent	Aud (persecution)	Possession, persecution reference	S.acute
2	M	21:5	1/3	–			Anxiety, irritation, autism		Depers		Reference	Acute
3	M	21:2	1/3	–			Monologue, inapp smile, strange behavior and words	Depressed mood		Aud (persecution)	Observation, reference	Acute
4	M	22:8	1/1	Unk			Excitement, hyperkinetic, wandering, monologue, inapp smile		Incoherent	Aud (content not clear)	Delusional mood	Acute
5	M	24:7	1/3	+			Abulia, autism, incoherence	Blunted feeling	Incoherent, thought broadcast		Delusional mood; persecution, reference	Acute
6	M	26:2	2/2	Unk	Hypobulia	1 m	Abnormal behaviors		Incoherent			Acute
7	F	20:6	1/1	+	Hypobulia	1 y	Abulia, autism	Labile mood	Thought deprivation	Aud (content not clear)		S.acute
8	F	22:8	3/3	+	Anxiety, irritation	1.5 y	Excitement, hyperkinetic, inapp smile, wandering	Blunted feeling				Latent
9	F	26:5	2/4	Unk			Monologue, inapp smile		Incoherent	Aud (content not clear)		S.acute
10	F	20:1	2/2	Unk						Aud (content not clear)	Persecution	Acute

Table 5. *Continued.*

Pt. no.	Sex	Age at onset[a]	Birth order/ siblings	Genetic factor	Prodromal symptoms Symptom	Onset	Abnormal behaviors	Abnormal moods	Main symptoms Thought disorders	Hallucinations	Delusions	Type of onset
Paranoid schizophrenia												
1	M	~21:0	1/2	+	Devoted to philosophy	3y	Violence		Thought broadcast	Aud	Persecution, reference	Latent
2	M	22:9	2/2	−			Wandering				Persecution (systematized)	Acute
3	M	26:7	2/2	−	Hypobulia	1y	Monologue, inapp smile		Thought broadcast, thought insertion	Aud	Persecution	S.acute
4	M	25:2	2/2	+			Monologue, inapp smile, wandering		Thought broadcast, easily influenced	Aud	Observation	Acute
5	M	26:6	2/3	−			Self-injury, monologue, inapp smile		Incoherent	Aud	Persecution, guilt	Acute
6	F	20:8	1/4	+					Thought broadcast, depers		Reference (systematized)	Acute
7	F	20:11	2/2	+	Attention disorder	7m	Obs-comp behaviors, violence, sexual acting out	Depressed mood	Obs-comp ideas	Aud	Persecution	S.acute
8	F	~23:0	3/3	−	Abulia, left job	1.5y	Monologue, inapp smile	Labile mood	Obs-comp ideas	Aud	Reference	Latent
9	F	24:1	1/1	−	Hypobulia	1m	Abulia, monologue	Depressed mood	Thought broadcast, depers	Aud	Persecution, reference	Acute
10	F	26:1	3/3	−	Hypobulia	2m		Depressed mood		Aud	Delusional loving; pregnacy (systematized)	Acute

See Table 3 for explanation of abbreviations. Also: Unk, unknown.
[a]Years:months.

group U were auditory hallucinations and delusions of persecution, reference, and possession. Moreover, other clinical symptoms of group U were irritability, instablity of their environmental or interpersonal relationships, and labile mood (nos. 2, 4, 6, 9, 10, 11, 14).

2. *Prodromal symptoms and types of onset*: There were six cases of latent-onset type and only one case of acute-onset type in group F, whereas there were five cases of acute-onset type and two cases each of subacute- and latent-onset types in group U.

3. *Personal history*: At birth, abnormalities or problems occurred in six patients (60%) of group F and in only one patient (11.1%) of group U. Six patients (60%) in group F and two patients (22.2%) in group U were physically ill until the age of 3 years. Concerning their adaptation during early childhood, all the patients of group F were isolated and played alone, whereas half of the patients of group U were relatively active and played with other children.

Analysis of Rorschach Test Data

Childhood Versus Adult Schizophrenia

Tables 6 and 7 show the Rorschach test data of group C. Tables 8 and 9 compare the Rorschach test data of groups C and A. F+% and A% were higher and deviant verbalizations were lower in group C than in group A. The content range was significantly narrower in group C than in group A.

Group F Versus Group U Versus Normal Children

Tables 10 and 11 show the Rorschach test results for groups F, U, and N (normal children). The fewest total responses were seen in group F and the most in group N, with significant differences between group F and group N. Group F had the most patients with Rejection and group N the fewest, with the difference being significant. Group F had the lowest F. L. A. value and group N the highest value, with significant differences between groups F and U and groups F and N. Group F had the highest F% value with significant differences between groups F and U and groups F and N. Group F had the lowest F+% value and group N the highest value, with significant differences between groups F and N and groups U and N. Group F had the lowest value for Popular reaction and group N the highest value, with significant differences between groups F and N and groups U and N. In the Content range, group F had the narrowest range and group N the widest range, with significant differences between groups F and U and groups F and N. Group F had the lowest value in Affect% and group N the highest value, with significant differences between groups F and U and groups U and N. Group N had the lowest value in Unpleasant%, with significant differences between groups U and N. Group F had the lowest value in Pleasant% and group N the highest value, with significant differences between groups F and N and groups U and N. Group U had the most cases of Deviant verbalization, with significant differences between groups F and N and groups U and N.

Discussion

Schizophrenia in children was clearly distinguished from infantile autism during the late 1970s and diagnosed in 1980s according to DSM-III criteria. The study presented in this chapter was carried out to clarify the characteristics of childhood schizophrenia based on the standardized diagnostic criteria, as described above.

Table 6. Rorschach test results from children with schizophrenia.

Pt. no.	Sex	R. test age	Total response	Rejection	Response time			F.L.A.	F%	F+%	M:FM
					Total	Achromatic	Chromatic				
1	M	10:6	12	0	27.0	23.8	30.2	0.1	100	25.0	0:0
2	M	13:8	11	0	12.4	9.6	15.2	0.9	45.4	60.0	1:3
3	M	14:7	24	0	18.6	14.2	25.0	0.7	83.3	90.0	0:1
4	M	14:3	11	0	11.3	13.4	9.2	0.8	54.5	66.7	2:1
5	M	14:5	14	0	10.4	10.4	10.4	1.0	50.0	85.7	2:2
6	M	15:2	18	0	9.7	11.2	8.2	1.0	50.0	77.8	0:8
7	M	15:0	9	IV, VII, IX, X	69.0	61.0	77.7	0.3	55.6	40.0	2:0
8	M	15:1	11	VII	28.8	21.0	35.2	0.6	100	81.8	0:0
9	F	12:0	29	0	15.1	10.2	20.0	0.6	44.7	38.3	1:5
10	F	13:1	21	IV, IX	4.8	3.3	6.3	1.1	66.7	76.4	2:1
11	F	14:3	20	0	5.6	7.8	3.4	1.1	50.0	80.0	4:2
12	F	13:6	8	II, VI, VII, IX	21.5	15.0	28.0	0.5	100	62.5	0:0
13	F	14:2	13	IX	4.1	5.6	2.6	0.7	92.3	83.3	0:0
14	F	15:1	19	0	7.9	7.6	8.2	0.9	57.8	81.8	3:4
15	F	14:7	9	II, IV	6.0	8.3	3.8	0.7	88.9	87.5	0:0
16	F	15:1	15	X	9.7	7.6	12.3	0.9	86.7	76.8	1:0
17	F	15:6	13	0	6.1	6.8	5.4	1.0	69.2	100	1:1
18	F	16:8	10	0	18.5	18.2	18.8	0.2	100	30.0	0:0
19	F	16:3	9	VI, VII, IX	12.1	11.5	13.0	1.1	33.3	100	3:2

Table 7. Rorschach test results of children with schizophrenia (continued).

Pt. no.	A%	H%	P	Content range	Affect %	Unpleasant %	Pleasant %	Deviant verbalization
1	83.3	0	1	2	83.3	100	0	1
2	81.8	9.0	3	7	63.6	100	0	4
3	70.8	8.3	4	2	13.3	100	0	1
4	54.5	27.2	4	4	18.2	100	0	0
5	57.1	21.4	3	5	28.6	50.0	50.0	0
6	88.9	5.0	4	3	33.3	100	0	1
7	33.8	33.3	0	4	33.3	66.7	33.3	1
8	45.4	9.0	2	3	27.2	33.3	66.7	0
9	34.4	3.4	3	9	37.9	63.6	36.4	3
10	57.1	19.0	2	5	23.8	60.0	40.0	1
11	50.0	30.0	3	4	30.0	50.0	50.0	0
12	100	22.2	5	3	33.3	66.7	33.3	0
13	46.1	53.8	2	2	7.7	100	0	0
14	42.1	36.8	4	5	42.1	25.0	75.0	0
15	66.7	22.2	5	3	33.3	66.7	33.3	0
16	86.7	26.6	4	2	13.3	100	0	1
17	76.9	23.1	6	2	0	0	0	1
18	90.0	0	0	2	40.0	75.0	25.0	2
19	44.4	33.3	2	5	44.4	25.0	75.0	1

Table 8. Rorschach test: comparison of results from children and adults.

Subject	Total response	Rejection +	Rejection −	Response time Total	Response time Achromatic	Response time Chromatic	F.L.A.	F%	F+%	M:FM M≥	M:FM M<
Children (n = 19)	14.5 (5.7)	8	11	15.7 (14.4)	14.0 (12.2)	17.5 (17.3)	0.7 (0.3)	69.9 (22.2)	70.7 (21.9)	6	5
Adults (n = 20)	16.5 (8.2)	10	10	13.5 (7.1)	12.3 (4.5)	14.8 (7.7)	0.7 (0.3)	60.0 (22.0)	58.3 (22.4)	9	7
t-Test	NS	NS[a]		NS	NS	NS	NS	NS	*	NS[a]	

NS, not significant.
[a] According to the chi-square test.
* <0.10.

Table 9. Rorschach test: comparison of results from children and adults (continued).

Subject	FC:CF+C FC≧	FC:CF+C FC<	P	A %	Content range	H%	Affect %	Unpleasant %	Pleasant %	Deviant verbalization
Children	6	8	2.8 (1.6)	63.6 (20.1)	3.8 (1.9)	19.0 (14.0)	29.9 (18.9)	64.0 (29.7)	25.5 (26.6)	0.8 (1.0)
Adults	2	11	2.8 (1.6)	53.1 (18.0)	5.5 (2.4)	19.5 (16.1)	25.6 (15.6)	61.0 (35.8)	23.9 (27.1)	2.0 (2.7)
t-Test	NS[a]		NS	*	**	NS	NS	NS	NS	*

NS, not significant.
[a] According to the chi-square test.
* <0.10; ** <0.05.

Clinical Features of Childhood Schizophrenia

Since Kydd and Werry [5], Eggers [6, 7], Goh [8], and others reported that the lower age limit for the onset of schizophrenia was about 8 to 10 years, the subjects described herein fulfilled their criteria. The male/female ratio was reported to be 25:32 by Eggers

Table 10. Rorschach test: comparison of results from two schizophrenic children groups and normal children.

Subjects	Total response	Rejection +	Rejection −	Response time Total	Response time achromatie	Response time Chromatie	F.L.A.	F%	F+%	M:FM M≥	M:FM M≤
Group F (n = 9)	12.4 (4.6)	6	3	20.2 (19.0)	17.6 (16.2)	23.2 (22.1)	0.65 (0.25)	86.2 (14.3)	72.4 (22.2)	3	1
Group U (n = 8)	16.5 (4.5)	2	6	10.4 (2.9)	9.6 (2.9)	11.3 (4.2)	0.93 (0.2)	50.3 (9.2)	73.4 (17.4)	4	4
Group N (n = 10)	18.1 3.9	1	9	18.3 (14.5)	15.9 (11.7)	21.8 (19.7)	1.03 (0.08)	54.4 (14.6)	94.5 (6.8)	4	6
t-Test											
F–U	1.75*	7.2***		NS	NS	NS	2.49**	4.76**	NS	NS[a]	
F–N	2.77**			NS	NS	NS	4.28**	4.53**	2.84**		
U–N	NS			NS	NS	NS	NS	NS	3.31**		

NS, not significant; group U, unstable schizophrenics; group F, flat schizophrenic group; group N, normal children.
[a] According to the chi-square test.
* <0.10; ** <0.05.

Table 11. Rorschach test: comparison of results from two schizophrenic children groups and normal children.

Subjects	FC:CF+C FC≥	FC:CF+C FC<	P	A%	Content range	H%	Affect %	Unpleasant %	Pleasant %	Deviant verbalization
Group F (n = 9)	5	1	2.8 (1.1)	68.4 (21.4)	2.7 (1.2)	19.6 (16.4)	18.1 (14.5)	60.2 (38.0)	17.6 (22.4)	0.6 (0.7)
Group U (n = 8)	1	6	3.1 (0.8)	57.5 (17.8)	5.4 (1.7)	19.4 (11.9)	36.5 (13.2)	65.4 (29.8)	34.6 (29.8)	1.2 (1.4)
Group N (n = 10)	5	3	4.7 (1.0)	55.9 (14.1)	4.8 (1.3)	23.9 (11.7)	18.6 (13.1)	34.0 (32.5)	56.0 (35.7)	0.1 (0.3)
t-Test										
F–U	6.7[a]		NS	NS	3.60**	NS	2.57**	NS	NS	NS
F–N			3.74**	NS	3.46**	NS	NS	NS	2.63**	4.74**
U–N			3.47**	NS	NS	NS	2.71**	1.99*	2.14**	2.28**

See Table 10 for explanation of abbreviations.
[a] According to the chi-square test.
* <0.10; ** <0.05.

[6] 8:7 by Kydd [5], and 52:48 by Goh [8]; in this study it was 8:11. Concerning the presence of genetic factors, Eggers [6, 7] reported that a genetic factor was found in 49.1%, Goh and Bose [8] in 29%, and Kydd and Werry [5] in 26.7%; it was about the same among my subjects (36.8%).

With regard to clinical symptoms, Eggers [6, 7] reported that after age 10 many patients with schizophrenia had delusions about religious and depressive subjects and about reference; and visual hallucinations were reported by half of the patients. Kolvin and Ounsted [3] reported that grimacing (63%), mannerisms (84%), deprivation of thoughts (20%), infusion of thoughts (20%), broadcasting of thoughts (20%), blocking of thoughts (60%), and blunted feelings (63%) were commonly observed. Among the various types of hallucination, auditory hallucination (81%) most commonly occurred, although cenesthesic hallucinations (36%) visual hallucinations (30%) were observed as well. Delusions of persecution (42%) and fantastic delusions (39%) were commonly observed. Goh and Bose [8] reported that the symptoms commonly seen with schizophrenia were auditory hallucinations (36%), visual hallucinations (8%), delusions (48%), monologues (51%), and inappropriate smiling (47%). Mannerisms, blunted feelings, blocked thoughts, and visual hallucinations were less commonly observed in my subjects than in those of Eggers [6, 7] and Kolvin and Ounsted [3]. Whereas in my subjects delusions of persecution (32%) and possession (15.8%) were reported, delusions of a religious theme were not seen as commonly as in the patients of Eggers [6, 7].

In this study, catatonic symptoms/signs occurred in two patients. Ando [9] reported that catatonic symptoms/signs occurred in 2 of his 15 patients; and Eggers [6, 7] reported two patients with catatonic stupor and one patients with hebe-catatonia among his group of 57 schizophrenic children. Hence catatonic symptoms/signs seem not to be common among schizophrenic children.

Eggers [6, 7] and Kydd and Werry [5] reported that half of the patients showed prodromal symptoms, and Ando [9] reported prodromal symptoms in 14 of 15 patients. Similarly, 15 of 19 of my subjects had prodromal symptoms. It is likely that many schizophrenic children have prodromal symptoms.

Regarding treatment, most of the patients required hospitalization and were administered high doses of a major tranquilizer. It was not always associated with the severity or the poor prognosis of childhood schizophrenia, however, considering my later study on prognosis.

Clinical features of Childhood and Adult Schizophrenia

Compared to the patients in group A, the clinical features of group C were characterized as follows: First, more first-born patients were observed in group C (73.7%) than in group A (40.0%). In view of the fact that there was only one child in some of the families in both groups (group C, 2 cases, 10.5%; group A, 3 cases, 15.0%) and the low average number of siblings (group C, 2.1; group A, 2.4), it is likely that childhood schizophrenia occurs in first-born children for several reasons (e.g., parental factors).

Second, more prodromal symptoms and cases of latent-onset schizophrenia were observed in group C. The age at which the prodromal symptoms presented (before the onset of schizophrenia) for patient 1 was 5 years 5 months, for patient 2 it was 11 years 4 months, for patient 3 it was about 11 years, for patient 7 it was about 11 years, for patient 12 it was 11 years 6 months, for patient 14 it was about 11 years, for patient 15 it was 12 years, and for patient 18 it was 14 years 10 months. Thus more patients gradually and latently develop symptoms of schizophrenia in group C, and prodromal symptoms (e.g., school refusal or violence) appeared at about age 11.

Third, visual hallucinations were more commonly observed in children than in adults. Fourth, patients in group C with auditory hallucinations were not able to describe their content as clearly as could the adult schizophrenics, and the duration of the hallucination was briefer. Fifth, none of group C had systematized delusions. Three patients (nos. 4, 11, 16) reported related themes in their delusions, but the content was simple.

Sixth, more children had labile moods, which became highly evident in their interpersonal relationships. Although they sought interpersonal relationships, because of their emotional instability they demonstrated ambivalence, dependence, resistance, or acting out, such as violence, running away from home, or suicide attempts. Finally obsessive compulsive symptoms were observed more often in children than adults.

Characteristics of Group F and Group U

Two patients (nos. 1 and 11) were excluded from the F/U classification because they demonstrated the catatonic syndrome. In group F most of the patients had had premorbid symptoms, such as school refusal, abnormal behaviors, or hypobulia for a long time, followed by schizophrenic symptoms. The main symptoms after the onset of childhood schizophrenia were gradual changes in character, abulia, and autism. Those negative symptoms developed slowly during the course of treatment. In five of the six patients who complained of auditory hallucinations, the contents were not described clearly, and the duration was brief. In terms of interpersonal relationships, most of the patients tended to be isolated.

In contrast, in group U most of the patients had no or a short premorbid period and had acute-onset schizophrenia. The main symptoms after the onset were delusions and hallucinations, but none of the patients had systematized delusions. Hallucinations occurred in all the patients ($n = 8$), and only three patients could not describe the contents clearly, with the duration of the hallucination brief. Most of the patients exhibited labile moods, which became particularly evident in their interpersonal relationships. Thus the characteristics of each group in this study fulfilled the criteria for childhood schizophrenia.

Analysis of Rorschach Test Data

Group C Versus Group A

The patients with childhood schizophrenia showed significantly higher values for F% and A% than the patients with adult schizophrenia. The children also had fewer words in Deviant verbalization and a narrower range in Content range, with the differences being significant. It is generally known that children have a higher A% value and a narrower range in Content range than adults. On the other hand, the higher F+% value and the lower Deviant verbalization value in group C reflected their clinical symptoms; that is, the contents of their auditory hallucinations were not explained clearly, and systematized delusions were not observed.

Group F Versus Group U Versus Normal Children

According to the analysis of the Rorschach test results, the patients in group F had poor psychic energies and flattened emotions. Although patients in group U did not have debilitated psychic energies, volition, or expanse of ideas, they had poor ability to understand reality and poor control of affect. These results confirm the clinical features of group F and group U, respectively.

Conclusions

Nineteen schizophrenic children who met the diagnostic criteria of DSM-III were investigated. The age of the patients at the onset of schizophrenia was less than 15 years. When the clinical features and Rorschach test results of the childhood schizophrenia group (group C) were compared with those of the adult schizophrenia group (group A), the following characteristics of child schizophrenia were noted. In terms of the clinical features: (1) More first-born patients were observed in group C. (2) More prodromal symptoms and latent-onset schizophrenia were found. (3) Some of the patients had visual hallucinations. (4) The contents of the auditory hallucinations were less clearly described, and the duration was briefer. (5) Few patients had systematized delusions. (6) Labile mood was more commonly observed in the children. (7) Most of the patients had obsessive compulsive symptoms.

The Rorschach test results revealed a lower value in deviant verbalization and more real descriptions for the young schizophrenics. The results reflected the clinical symptoms/signs of group C; that is, the contents of the auditory hallucinations were less clearly described, and systematized delusions were not observed.

The patients with childhood schizophrenia were then classified according to their main clinical symptoms after the onset of schizophrenia. Two groups emerged: a flat group and an unstable group. The main clinical symptoms of the flat group were gradual changes in character, abulia, and autism. In contrast, those of the unstable group were hallucinations and delusions. The symptoms of each group were related to the type of onset of their schizophrenia; for instance, group was F related to a latent onset, and group U was related to an acute onset.

According to the analysis of the Rorschach test results, the patients of group F had poor psychic energies and flattened emotions. In contrast, the patients of group U did not have debilitated psychic energies, volition, or expanse of ideas; but they were only poorly able to understand reality and had poor control over their affect. These results correlate with the clinical features of group F and group U.

References

1. Rutter M, Lockyer L (1967) A five to fifteen year follow-up study of infantile psychosis. A. Description of sample. Br J Psychiatry 113:1169–1182
2. Rutter M, Greenfield D, Lockyer L (1967) A five to fifteen year follow-up study of infantile psychosis. B. Social and behavioral outcome. Br J Psychiatry 113:1183–1199
3. Kolvin I, Ounsted C (1971) Studies in childhood psychoses. Br J Psychiatry 118:381–419
4. American Psychiatric Association (1980) Diagnostic and statistical manual of mental disorders (DSM-III). American Psychiatric Association, Washington, DC
5. Kydd RR, Werry JS (1982) Schizophrenia in children under 16 years. J Autism Dev Disord 12:343–357
6. Eggers C (1978) Course and prognosis of childhood schizophrenia. J Autism Child Schizoph 8:21–36
7. Eggers C (1982) Psychosis in childhood and adolescence. Acta Paedopsychiatr ••:81–98
8. Goh CW Bose P (1979) a clinical profile of 100 child-patients with schizophrenia. Ann •• Acad Med 8:252–261
9. Ando K (1985) Schizophrenia in childhood. Seishin Igaku [Clinical Psychiatry] 27:1255–1266

Depressive Disorder During Childhood and Adolescence in Japan

Toyohisa Murata[1], Yoko Sarada[2], Tatsuki Tsutsumi[3], Youichi Nakaniwa[2], and Yuuki Shinpo[2]

Summary. The aim of this study was to investigate the depressive condition among normal children and adolescents as well as psychiatric outpatient children. We have used the Children's Depression Inventory (CDI) because this index has been most commonly cited and thoroughly researched. The psychiatric clinic-referred patients comprised 86 "depressed" and 181 "nondepressed" children 7–15 years old. The mean CDI score of the depressed group was 26.4 ± 7.02 and that of the nondepressed group 16.5 ± 7.97. The cutoff score for the CDI in Japanese juveniles was determined to be 22. The normal subjects (controls) were 1041 elementary school children (537 boys, 504 girls) in grades 2–6 and 543 junior high school adolescents (274 boys, 269 girls), ranging in age from 12 to 15 years. The mean CDI score of the elementary school children was 14.2 ± 6.90, and 13.3% of these children had a score higher than the cutoff score of 22. The mean CDI score of junior high school adolescents was 16.5 ± 7.60, with 21.9% higher than the cutoff score of 22. In both psychiatric and normal groups, Japanese children were found to be fairly depressed.

Key words. Depressive disorder—Childhood—Adolescence—Children's Depression Inventory—Prevalence

Introduction

Until recently in Japan the concept that children could be depressed was not widely recognized, but since the mid-1980s it has received increased attention. The diagnostic category and explanation of the *DSM-III-R* has helped to increase attention to this term. Therefore Japanese child psychiatrists have begun to accept the existence of depression in children and have diagnosed depression even in those as young as 8–10 years.

---

[1] Department of Educational Psychology, Faculty of Education, Kyushu University, 6-19-1 Hakozaki, Higashi-ku, Fukuoka-shi 812, Japan
[2] Department of Psychiatry, Fukuoka University, School of Medicine, 7-45-1 Nanakuma, Jonan-ku, Fukuoka-shi 814-80, Japan
[3] Tsutsumi Kokura Hospital, 358 Horikoshi, Kokuraminami-Ku, Kitakyushu-shi 802, Japan

The prevalence and frequency of depressive disorder during childhood and adolescence have not been systematically investigated. Although many children are now being diagnosed as suffering from depression in Japan, its incidence among clinically referred patients and the prevalence of depressive disorder in the normal population have not been clarified [1]. Therefore we wished to study the prevalence of depressive symptomatology among normal subjects as well as psychiatric outpatient children using an instrument that measures a broad spectrum of childhood depressive conditions.

Method

Although a variety of rating scales have been developed in attempts to obtain consistent, reliable data on the depressive condition [2], the most thoroughly investigated and frequently used self-report measure is the Children's Depression Inventory (CDI). The CDI was developed by Kovacs as a downward revision and modification of the 21-item Beck Depression Inventory [3]. The current CDI version consists of 27 items. Each of these 27 items is composed of three statements that are graded in severity and assigned numerical values from 0 to 2, providing a total score of 0 to 54. We adopted the CDI and performed the Japanese version of this inventory [4] with permission of Professor Kovacs.

The purposes of this study were twofold: (1) to discover how well the CDI discriminates clinically diagnosed depressed from nondepressed outpatients and to find the most useful cutoff point; and (2) to examine the prevalence of depressive symptomatology in an adequate number of samples of elementary school children and junior high school adolescents using the CDI.

Results

Table 1 shows CDI mean scores for clinically referred patients. For prepubertal children (elementary school boys and girls 8–12 years of age) the CDI mean score for 41 depressed children was 26.4 and that for 99 nondepressed children 16.5. Among adolescents (junior high school students 12–15 years of age), the CDI mean score for 45 depressed youths was 27.2 and for 82 nondepressed youths 17.5. These results clearly demonstrate that there were large differences in the CDI mean scores between the depressed group and the nondepressed group. It also means that the CDI can be properly used in the clinical setting to clearly distinguish depressed from nondepressed psychiatric child outpatients in Japan.

Table 1. CDI mean scores for children and adolescents.

Subjects	CDI score (mean ± SD)	P
Children		
Depressed ($n = 41$)	26.40 ± 7.02	
Not depressed ($n = 99$)	16.50 ± 7.97	<0.01
Adolescents		
Depressed ($n = 45$)	27.20 ± 7.90	
Not depressed ($n = 82$)	17.50 ± 6.63	<0.01

CDI, Children's Depression Inventory.

To determine the cutoff point that best discriminates depressed from nondepressed groups, a characteristic analysis was performed. As Table 2 displays, a cutoff score of 22 was the most significant of three tested and gave a sensitivity of 78.0%, a specificity of 77.8%, and a misclassification rate of 22.2%. The CDI cutoff score in Japanese juveniles was therefore set at 22, although this score is higher than that for children in the United States and Canada. In 1982 Kovacs proposed a score of 12 as useful for detecting depressed subjects [3]. Six years later in 1988 Costello and Angold recom-

Table 2. Usefulness of three empirically derived CDI cutoff scores to identify diagnosed depressed and nondepressed patients.

CDI cutoff	Sensibility (%) (true + rate)	Specificity (%) (true − rate)	Misclassified (%)
21	80.5	73.7	26.3
22	78.0	77.8	22.2
23	70.7	78.8	21.3

CDI, Children's Depression Inventory.

Table 3. Mean scores of each CDI item in a clinical population.

CDI item	Depressed disorder, mean ± SD ($n = 45$)	Nondepressed emotional disorder, mean ± SD ($n = 82$)	Significance
1. Sadness	0.78 ± 0.77	0.29 ± 0.60	**
2. Hopelessness	1.27 ± 0.65	1.05 ± 0.54	*
3. Self-depreciation	1.16 ± 0.60	0.83 ± 0.56	**
4. Anhedonia	1.11 ± 0.53	0.92 ± 0.45	*
5. Acting bad	0.62 ± 0.61	0.39 ± 0.60	*
6. Pessimistic worrying	1.09 ± 0.70	0.61 ± 0.71	**
7. Self-hate	1.42 ± 0.58	0.72 ± 0.69	**
8. Self-blame	0.96 ± 0.64	0.75 ± 0.64	*
9. Suicidal ideation	0.93 ± 0.62	0.52 ± 0.57	**
10. Crying	0.69 ± 0.73	0.22 ± 0.52	**
11. Feeling bothered	1.09 ± 0.79	0.67 ± 0.80	**
12. Socialization	0.67 ± 0.56	0.34 ± 0.57	**
13. Indecisiveness	1.13 ± 0.55	0.89 ± 0.61	
14. Negative body image	1.24 ± 0.65	0.95 ± 0.58	**
15. Reduced motivation for school work	1.38 ± 0.72	1.12 ± 0.77	*
16. Insomnia	0.78 ± 0.70	0.67 ± 0.73	
17. Tiredness	0.98 ± 0.72	0.66 ± 0.72	*
18. Reduced appetite	0.76 ± 0.68	0.39 ± 0.60	**
19. Somatic concerns	1.07 ± 0.75	0.75 ± 0.73	*
20. Loneliness	0.84 ± 0.71	0.31 ± 0.56	**
21. Fun at school	0.96 ± 0.60	0.60 ± 0.70	**
22. Social isolation	1.02 ± 0.62	0.63 ± 0.68	**
23. Decline in schoolwork	1.27 ± 0.65	0.83 ± 0.70	**
24. Self-comparison	1.36 ± 0.68	0.88 ± 0.77	**
25. Feeling unloved	1.11 ± 0.61	0.70 ± 0.56	**
26. Disobedience	0.89 ± 0.49	0.60 ± 0.56	**
27. Social problem	0.67 ± 0.71	0.22 ± 0.47	**

CDI, Children's Depression Inventory.
**$P < 0.01$; *$P < 0.05$.

Table 4. Children's Depression Inventory: mean scores for age groups and genders.

Grade	Female		Male		Both	
	No.	Mean ± SD	No.	Mean ± SD	No.	Mean ± SD
Elementary school						
Second	80	12.0 ± 6.10	75	14.3 ± 6.38	155	13.1 ± 6.10
Third	107	12.6 ± 6.81	122	12.6 ± 5.45	229	12.6 ± 6.12
Fourth	108	15.5 ± 7.57	106	14.5 ± 6.77	214	15.0 ± 7.20
Fifth	111	13.6 ± 6.32	116	14.0 ± 6.69	227	13.8 ± 6.51
Sixth	98	17.2 ± 7.66	118	15.3 ± 7.59	216	16.2 ± 7.68
Total	504	14.3 ± 7.13	537	14.1 ± 6.68	1041	14.2 ± 7.68
Junior high school						
Seventh	76	16.8 ± 7.40	87	13.9 ± 6.28	163	15.3 ± 6.95
Eighth	101	17.8 ± 6.79	91	16.2 ± 7.17	192	17.0 ± 7.00
Ninth	92	17.4 ± 8.48	96	16.7 ± 8.67	188	17.1 ± 8.56
Total	269	17.4 ± 7.56	274	15.7 ± 7.55	543	16.5 ± 7.60

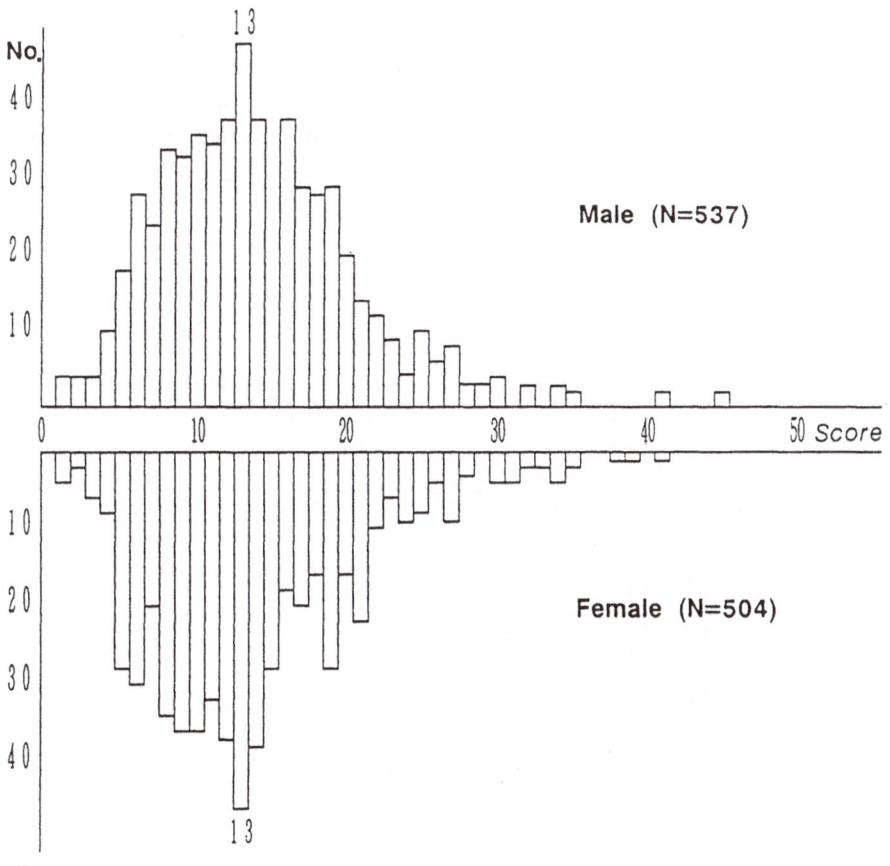

Fig. 1. Children's Depression Inventory score distribution for a nonclinical population (children from three elementary schools, second to sixth grade).

mended that 18 be the cutoff point for contemporary children [5]. This difference between those two countries and Japan seems to be meaningful.

We next investigated the mean item scores on the CDI for psychiatric out-patients at junior high school ages. As Table 3 shows, the depressed group had higher mean scores on all items. Most items, except item 13 (indecisiveness) and item 16 (insomnia), are statistically significantly different for the two groups.

The next phase was to study the prevalence of depression in the general population. Our normal group was composed of 1041 elementary school children (grades 2–6) from three schools in Fukuoka Prefecture and 543 junior high school students (grades 7–9) from two schools in the same area.

For elementary school children, the mean total CDI score was 14.2 with a standard deviation of 7.68; 13.3% of these children scored higher than the cutoff score of 22 (Table 4). Figure 1 displays the CDI score distributions for the younger children. The two groups (boys and girls) had a normal caussian distribution.

For junior high school students, the mean total CDI score was 16.5 with a standard deviation of 7.60; 21.9% scored higher than the cutoff score of 22 (Table 4). Figure 2 displays the CDI score distributions for the junior high school students. The distribution curves for these students are somewhat different from those for the elementary school students, especially for the female students, for whom two peaks are shown. It was surprising that the mean total CDI scores were higher than those obtained for American children and adolescents [6].

Table 4 shows age- and gender-related differences in the mean total scores. The female subjects tended to have higher CDI mean scores than male subjects, with this gender difference becoming more prominent in the junior high school groups. Large

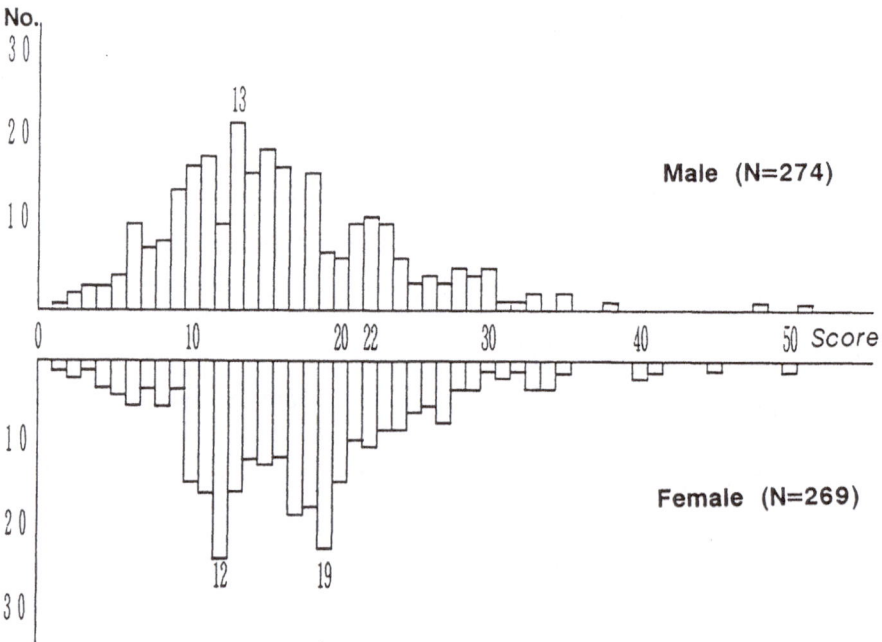

Fig. 2. Children's Depression Inventory score distribution for a nonclinical population (juveniles from two junior high schools, seventh to ninth grade).

gender differences were not observed in the preadolescent children. This trend suggests that the study of depression should take developmental level and gender into account.

Table 5 shows a gender comparison of the mean scores of each CDI item for the junior high school students. A negative view of self (negative body image, self-hate) and a general dysphoric mood (sadness, loneliness, crying) correlated more highly for the adolescent girls than for the same-age boys. This finding suggests that female adolescents tend to internalize depression at an earlier age than do the same-age boys, and they are more likely to manifest internally focused characteristics.

The next step of the study was to investigate whether there were differences in the contents of depressive symptomatology in the depressed clinically referred patients and high CDI score subjects from the general population (nonclinical group). For this purpose, a factor analysis was carried out for the clinically referred depressed group and the high-CDI nonclinical group to determine if there might be any characteristics that would provide better discrimination. For this procedure the subjects were limited to junior high school juveniles. Four factors emerged. Table 6 demonstrates the differences between these two groups. In both groups five items were

Table 5. Mean scores of each item of the CDI according to gender (nonclinical population: 543 junior high school juveniles).

CDI item	Female, mean ± SD ($n = 269$)	Male, Mean ± SD ($m = 274$)	P
1. Sadness	0.24 ± 0.51	0.16 ± 0.26	<0.01
2. Hopelessness	1.06 ± 0.53	0.91 ± 0.35	<0.05
3. Self-depreciation	0.77 ± 0.56	0.69 ± 0.32	
4. Anhedonia	0.60 ± 0.54	0.74 ± 0.20	
5. Acting bad	0.34 ± 0.59	0.37 ± 0.64	
6. Pessimistic worrying	0.62 ± 0.74	0.65 ± 0.75	
7. Self-hate	0.98 ± 0.64	0.58 ± 0.68	<0.01
8. Self-blame	0.84 ± 0.59	0.81 ± 0.63	
9. Suicidal ideation	0.71 ± 0.58	0.42 ± 0.60	<0.01
10. Crying	0.27 ± 0.56	0.15 ± 0.48	<0.01
11. Feeling bothered	0.55 ± 0.76	0.50 ± 0.78	
12. Socialization	0.14 ± 0.39	0.15 ± 0.41	
13. Indecisiveness	1.00 ± 0.59	0.92 ± 0.64	
14. Negative body image	1.08 ± 0.58	0.86 ± 0.57	<0.01
15. Reduced motivation for school work	1.16 ± 0.75	1.11 ± 0.78	
16. Insomnia	0.36 ± 0.27	0.39 ± 0.63	
17. Tiredness	0.80 ± 0.73	0.91 ± 0.77	
18. Reduced appetite	0.26 ± 0.52	0.27 ± 0.53	
19. Somatic concerns	0.62 ± 0.71	0.44 ± 0.68	
20. Loneliness	0.31 ± 0.55	0.23 ± 0.52	
21. Fun at school	0.47 ± 0.59	0.52 ± 0.64	
22. Social isolation	0.46 ± 0.54	0.36 ± 0.54	
23. Decline in schoolwork	0.84 ± 0.68	0.88 ± 0.75	
24. Self-comparison	1.09 ± 0.71	0.96 ± 0.73	
25. Feeling unloved	0.94 ± 0.49	0.90 ± 0.54	
26. Disobedience	0.58 ± 0.53	0.67 ± 0.56	
27. Social problem	0.26 ± 0.50	0.23 ± 0.50	

CDI, Children's Depression Inventory.

Table 6. Factor analysis on the CDI items: varimax analysis.

Clinically referred depressed group[a]	High-CDI-score group in nonclinical sample[b]
Factor 1[a]	
Feel like crying	Feel like crying
Sadness	Sadness
Feel bothered	Feel bothered
Hopelessness	Pessimistic worrying
Persevere at school	Suicidal ideation
Factor 2	
Negative body image	Loneliness
Self-comparison	Social withdrawal
Feels he/she is bad	Lack of friendships
Feels unloved	Lack of fun at school
Factor 3	
Social withdrawal	Hopelessness
Self-blame	Feels bothered
Loneliness	Self-hate
Pessimistic worrying	
Self-depreciation	
Factor 4	
Insomnia	Reduced appetite
Anhedonia	Fatigue
Feels bothered	Insomnia
Fatigue	
Reduced appetite	

CDI, Children's Depression Inventory.
[a]Percent variance for factors 1, 2, 3, and 4 were 24.0%, 14.6%, 10.9%, and 8.9%, respectively.
[b]Percent variance for factors 1, 2, 3, and 4 were 17.6%, 8.2%, 6.8%, and 6.4%, respectively.

loaded for factor 1. They centered around "sadness." The results were similar for the two groups.

The results for factor 2 show definite differences. Four items were loaded that focused on interpersonal relationships, although the items were of a different nature for the two groups. For the depressed group, the four items seem to stand for "negative self-image," whereas for the nonclinical group the items suggested "isolation." These differences seem meaningful.

Factor 3 also reveals differences between the groups. First, five items were loaded for the depressed group in contrast to three items for the nonclinical group. Second, the items for the depressed group signified a lower self-image with a tendency to withdrawal than those for the high-score nonclinical group.

Factor 4 was concerned mainly with "somatic symptoms," and there was a clear difference between the two groups. For the depressed group, the items "anhedonia" and "feels bothered" were added to three somatic items.

The investigation of this factor analysis brought us to the conclusion that these two group were composed of fairly different subjects. Hence further investigation is required to determine the supposed prevalence rate of depression in the general population of children and adolescents.

Table 7. Multivariance discriminant analysis on the CDI items.

Patient group	Diagnosis of depression	
	Reliable (%)	Uncertain (%)
Clinically referred depressed group ($n = 45$)	68.9	31.1
High-CDI-score group in nonclinical sample ($n = 119$)	26.9	73.1

CDI, Children's Depression Inventory.

A popular tool for discrimination purposes is the multivariance discriminant analysis. Table 7 shows the results of this analysis for the two groups. Multivariance discriminant analysis on the CDI items proved that 26.9% of the high-scoring group of the nonclinical population could be assigned a diagnosis of depression as defined by the CDI, whereas 68.9% of the clinically referred depressed group fulfilled this criterion.

Discussion

It is now possible to speculate on the prevalence of depressive disorder in Japanese junior high school students (ages 12–15). In our study 21.9% of students in the general population exceeded the CDI cutoff score of 22, and 26.9% of these high-CDI-score subjects proved to be truly depressive by multivariance discriminant analysis. It is possible to compose an equation as follows: $0.219 \times 0.269 \times 100 = 5.89\%$. With this equation the supposed prevalence rate is 5.89%.

It is surprising to discover this 5.89% rate, which is fairly high when compared with the prevalence rate for American and European children [7–9]. Because we have used the *DSM-III-R* criteria and the American self-rating instrument, the high rate is probably not due to our clinical criteria or diagnostic methods.

Why, then, were the CDI scores for Japanese children so high? There appear to be two reasons. First, various types of stress in the Japanese educational situation must be noted. In elementary and junior high schools, academic training is the focus of education. Value systems in the family and the society have a tendency to be influenced by the results of this academic work. These tendencies have tended to produce children with narrow values and somewhat neurotic pessimistic traits [10].

Second, it is important to consider the characteristics of cognitive function of Japanese children. Studies on the Morita syndrome (a form of anthropophobia found in Japanese culture) during childhood have shown that Japanese children have a tendency to develop introspective functioning and feelings of self-insufficiency. As a consequence, self-awareness at a cognitive level and self-depreciation are developed from early childhood. It is possible that Japanese children are less suspicious of the CDI items, many of which reflect social cognitive problems [1]. Our study of depressed children using CDI has proved to be helpful for clarifying the psychological characteristics of the present-day Japanese children in the general population. We think it worthwhile to continue this line of study.

References

1. Sarada Y, Murata T (1992) Depression in childhood (in Japanese). Jpn J Psychiatr Treat 7:833–840
2. Kazdin AE (1990) Childhood depression. J Child Psychol Psychiatry 31:121–160

3. Kovacs M (1982) The Children's Depression Inventory. Unpublished manuscript, University of Pittsburgh
4. Murata T, Tsutsumi T, Sarada Y, Nakaniwa Y (1992) The validity and reliability of the Children's Depression Inventory—Japanese version (in Japanese). Kyushu N-psych 38:42–47
5. Costello EJ, Angold A (1988) Scales to assess child and adolescent depression: checklists, screens, and nets. J Am Acad Child Adolesc Psychiatry 27:726–737
6. Nelson WA, Poliano PM, Finch AJ, Wendel N, Mayhall C (1987) Children's Depression Inventory: normative data and utility with emotionally disturbed children. J Am Acad Child Adolesc Psychiatry 26:43–48
7. Harrington R (1993) Depressive disorder in childhood and adolescence. Wiley, New York, pp 65–83
8. Kandel DV, Davies M (1982) Epidemiology of depressive mood in adolescents. Arch Gen Psychiatry 43:255–262
9. Kashani JH, Simonds JF (1979) The incidence of depression in children. Am J Psychiatry 136:1203–1205
10. Murata T (1994) Adolescent depressive condition in Japan—from the viewpiont of Shimoda's theory (in Japanese). Jpn J Adolesc Psychiatry 42:142–151

Part 6

Other Fundamental Problems

Psychiatric Problems of Living Kidney Transplantation in Child and Adolescent Recipients

Kiichiro Sato, Keiko Akahoshi, Yasuyo Suzuki, Yoshitsuna Fukuyama, Akihiko Isomoto, and Sadanori Miura

Summary. A psychiatric follow-up study on child and adolescent patients who had living kidney transplantation donated from their close relatives at the Kitasato University Hospital is reported. There were 32 recipients ranging in age from 4 to 17 years (mean 11.4 years). The psychiatric states of the patients were studied at three stages, the periods of time relative to the transplantation procedure: (1) Just before transplantation. Commonly observed at this point was strong mutual child-mother binding, and most of the recipients tended to have emotionally and socially immature personalities. No recipients exhibited marked psychiatric symptoms. (2) Less than 4 years after transplantation. Various psychiatric problems were observed in 21 (65.6%) of the 32 recipients. The notable feature, which was markedly different from those reported in adult recipients, was that nearly half the patients exhibited a regressive state and a symbiotic relationship with their mothers. (3) More than 4 years after transplantation. Most recipients were unable to enjoy their new lives because of increasing fear of rejection reactions, with some suffering the Damocles syndrome. Eighteen (60%) of the 30 surviving recipients exhibited various psychiatric problems, such as dependency/withdrawal, depression, body-image disturbance, identity disorder with maladjustment to school life, and personality disorder. Based on these results, the psychiatric characteristics and their underlying mechanisms in young transplant recipients are discussed.

Key words. Kidney transplantation—Psychiatric problem—Child and adolescent recipients—Donor selection

Introduction

With recent advances in the development of immunosuppressant medications, treatment results of organ transplantation have markedly improved. In particular, many end-stage uremic patients have received great benefit from kidney transplantation. In the case of living related donor transplants, the current 1-year graft survival rate at the Kitasato University Hospital (KUH) is nearly 100%.

Department of Psychiatry, Kitasato University School of Medicine, 1-15-1 Kitasato, Sagamihara, Kanagawa 226, Japan

In Japan, the main source of transplantable kidneys is the family of the recipient, as the concept of cadaveric organ donation from brain-dead individuals is not yet well accepted. Accordingly, psychological problems among not only recipients but also donors are of particular interest. We have become especially interested in young transplant patients with special reference to the child's developmental processes.

We have been investigating the psychological problems with kidney transplantation at the KUH since 1972 [1–6]. This report describes some of the results obtained during the course of a psychiatric follow-up study of child and adolescent transplant recipients with special reference to their developmental processes.

Subjects and Procedure

Thirty-two recipients who were referred to the Kidney Center of the KUH for living donor kidney transplantation between 1972 and 1984 took part in the study. The recipients (16 boys, 16 girls) ranged in age from 4 to 17 years (mean 11.4 years) at the time of the transplant. The mean duration of illness before transplantation was 3.9 years, including 1.2-year hemodialysis period. For 24 (75%) patients the mother acted as donor (Table 1). At the time of this survey (1988) the interval after transplantaion ranged from 4 to 15 years (mean 8.1 years), and the survival rate of the grafts was 46.9% (15 of 32 recipients). The grafted kidneys of 11 recipients had been removed because of rejection; two of these patients died before the 1988 (final) portion of the survey.

At the KUH, all candidate donors and recipients undergo a psychiatric interview and psychological testing. For those with psychiatric or ethical problems, the transplantation procedures are stopped or suspended. For those who proceed to transplantation a psychiatric follow-up interview (and psychiatric intervention if necessary) is carried out occasionally (or regularly if needed).

In the present study, the psychiatric states of all patients were investigated and the periods they were followed were categorized into three stages: (1) just before transplantation; (2) less than 4 years after transplantation; and (3) more than 4 years after transplantation.

Table 1. Recipient-donor relationship.

Subjects	Mother donor	Father donor	Total
Age 4–6 years	5	2	7
Male	3	0	3
Female	2	2	4
Age 7–12 years	10	2	12
Male	4	1	5
Female	6	1	7
Age 13–17 years	9	4	13
Male	6	2	8
Female	3	2[a]	5
Total	24	8	32
Male	13	3	16
Female	11	5[a]	16

[a] One older brother.

Results

Recipient-Donor Considerations

As shown in Table 1, the donor was the mother in 24 cases (75%), the father in 7 cases (22%), and an older brother in 1 case (3%). Donor selection was smoother for child recipients and subsequent family problems were fewer, compared with adult recipients. Also, mothers reached their decision to donate much more quickly for child recipients compared with adult recipients. The majority of mothers had accepted the possibility that they might have to donate a kidney soon after the child began to dialyze. They tended to give the go-ahead for transplantation when they feared for their child's life or thought that delay might cause the child's condition to worsen, or when the child's school performance was deteriorating. Other family members made the decision to donate only in cases where it was impossible for the mother to become a donor due to physical or immunological considerations.

The motivations of the maternal donors were complex, with their true intentions often camouflaged or unconscious. In almost all cases, the motivation stated at the first interview was different from their actual intention, which we learned later. Often the mother's true motivation came to the fore during an episode when their child recipient was being treated for rejection of the kidney or for other complications.

The attitude of the mother was quite different from that of other family member donors. The mother's decision to become a donor was based on her emotional reaction to the child's suffering. The father's decision, on the other hand, was based on his wanting to restore his whole family to health and to re-create a healthy family life.

Psychiatric Problems Before Transplantation

After a child began dialysis, the parents often feared the death of the child and felt guilt over the development of the illness. They then tended to compensate for their fears by becoming overly protective and stressing the child's safety. These actions resulted in strict control over the child's behavior, which meant that the child had fewer chances of having real life experiences with his or her peers and thus developed few communication skills—in addition to growth disturbances due to the renal failure. The children under 10 years of age were immature socially and emotionally, and they exhibited deficient verbal expression and coping abilities compared to the extent of their actual knowledge. Therefore the longer the period of the renal disease in the child, the greater was the negative influence of the mother, whose pity for the subject, her own guilt, and her fear that the disease would get worse made her overly protective.

Twenty recipients were markedly immature emotionally and socially; they were regressive, dependent, shy, retiring, and egocentric, and they avoided communicating with their peers. These characteristics were more evident in the recipients whose disease had had an early onset or who had led shortened healthy lives. We found only nine recipients who were mentally healthy prior to transplantation. However, none was in a delirious state, and none had moderate or severe depression before transplantation. There were, though, several children in regressive and withdrawal states. In addition, 11 recipients had already become involved in a symbiotic relationship with their mothers.

Psychiatric Problems After Transplantation

At Three Years

By the fourth year after transplantation, we had observed various psychiatric problems in 21 recipients (65.6%) (Table 2). The incidence of such problems was higher than that reported for adults who had received a living donor transplant but lower than that for adults who had been given an organ from a cadaver; notably, the incidence was similar to that for the early mixed cases (mixed age group) reported in 1978 (45/70; 64.3%) [2]. The types of disorder, however, were different from those seen in adults and varied according to the age of onset and the postoperative course.

The most striking difference between the disorders in the children and those in adults was the high incidence of a symbiotic relationship with the mother and a regressive state of the child, which were observed in 14 subjects (43.8% of recipients, 58.3% of mother donors). Of these 14 subjects, 11 had been deemed regressive before transplantation, whereas 3 showed these characteristics only after transplantation. Although most of these children had become less regressive within a year, the six who experienced repeated rejections of the graft or other complications remained regressive longer. They were treated carefully so as to prevent more severe psychiatric problems until the time their parents demanded that they be, or that they were already, independent.

A delirious state was not seen in any of the subjects despite the fact that they had been given high-dosage steroids. Depression was observed in three subjects (9.4%). Two were older than 16 years; the third child was a 14-year-old girl whose depression was induced by steroids after a brief episode of hypomania. Two of the subjects who were treated unsuccessfully for 2 months were considered to have reactive depression. Their depression at this point of the study was milder than their depression after 4 years.

Marked dependence and withdrawal were observed in four recipients (12.5%) after recovery from severe rejection. These children were excessively dependent on their mother donors and avoided any social life except during school.

Marked anxiety and hypochondriasis were observed in four recipients (12.5%) during hospitalization for severe rejection. We believe that their state was induced by their mothers' anxiety, as they themselves had little anticipatory fear of death or rejection.

Conversion hysteria was seen in one girl. She feared loss of her mother and described her fear of abandonment by her mother after a second severe rejection episode.

Marked body image disturbances were observed in five recipients (15.6%: two boys, three girls). They suffered from cushingoid symptoms (especially moon face and obesity) and had not adjusted well to their school life. They experienced difficulty communicating with new classmates after entrance to high school. Two had strange sensations in their skin and had an operation scar, and three showed the Siamese-twins effect [7].

Marked maladjustment to school was seen in three recipients who had low IQs and who had been maladjusted even before transplantation. Their problems became marked after unsuccessful transplantation.

A sexual identity disorder was seen in a boy who was exhibiting female behavior, similar to that of his mother.

Table 2. Data from the study.

Pt. no.	Sex	Age at Tx	Dnor[a]	Age at the study	Year of Tx	Psychiatric problem		Personality disorder[d]	State of therapy[e]	Adjustment state at time of study
						Within 3 years[c]	After 4 years			
1 (T.M.)	M	5	Mo	20	1973	Rg-Damo	BID-ID-Damo		HD	Poor
2 (T.I.)	M	10	Mo	25	1973	STE-Rg-BID	BID-MA-Damo-X?	APD		Worse
3 (H.O.)	M	7	Mo	22	1974	STE-Rg-ANX	BID-MA-ID-Damo	DPD	HD	Worse
4 (F.M.)	F	13	Mo	(18)[b]	1974	Rg-ID (sex)	ID (sex)-Damo		D	—
5 (M.N.)	M	17	Br	30	1974					Excellent
6 (E.U.)	F	6	Mo	19	1975	Rg		BPD		Excellent
7 (E.M.)	F	16	Mo	28	1975	STE-Rg-HY-DW	ANX-Dep	DPD	HD	Poor
8 (T.S.)	F	16	Fa	28	1976	Dep			HD	Excellent
9 (E.Y.)	M	15	Fa	27	1976	MA-BID	MA-ID-X	APD	HD	Worse
10 (R.Y.)	M	13	Mo	24	1977					Excellent
11 (Y.S.)	F	12	Mo	23	1977	Rg				Excellent
12 (M.E.)	M	11	Fa	22	1978	Rg	ANX-Damo			Good
13 (H.T.)	M	13	Mo	24	1978	Rg-ANX-DW	HY-ANX	DPD	HD	Worse
14 (S.O.)	M	9	Mo	19	1978	Rg	BID-ANX-Damo			Good
15 (S.T.)	M	11	Mo	21	1978	Rg-ANX-Damo	DW-Dep	DPD	HD	Worse
16 (K.A.)	F	10	Mo	20	1978					Excellent
17 (A.M.)	F	5	Fa	14	1979		BID-MA-X		HD	Worse

18 (Y.S.)	F	5	Mo	14	1979	Rg-MA	Rg-MA		HD	Worse
19 (T.M.)	M	8	Mo	17	1980	Rg	BID-MA-Damo	DPD	D	Poor
20 (F.K.)	F	11	Mo	(18)[b]	1980	Rg	BID-MA-DW-Dep			—
21 (M.O.)	F	6	Fa	14	1980		Damo			Good
22 (K.A.)	M	12	Mo	20	1980	Rg-MA	Rg-MA-BID/ID-X	APD	HD	Worse
23 (T.S.)	M	14	Mo	21	1981	Rg	BID-ID-Damo			Good
24 (S.M.)	F	12	Mo	20	1981					Excellent
25 (A.F.)	F	13	Mo	21	1981	Rg-DW	BID-ID-MA-X?	DPD	HD	Worse
26 (M.E.)	F	8	Fa	(11)[b]	1981	BID	—		D	—
27 (S.A.)	M	17	Mo	24	1981	Rg-BID	BID-Damo			Good
28 (H.O.)	F	11	Mo	(13)[b]	1982	Rg-BID	—		D	—
29 (M.K.)	F	12	Mo	17	1982	Rg-M/Dep	BID-MA-ID	DPD	HD	Worse
30 (N.Y.)	M	16	Mo	21	1983	Dep-ANX	ANX-ID	DPD	HD	Worse
31 (E.Y.)	M	16	Fa	20	1984	Rg-ANX	ANX-Damo			Good
32 (Y.H.)	M	5	Mo	8	1984	Rg-ANX	ANX-Damo			Good

[a] Mo, mother; Fa, father; Br, brother.

[b] Age at death.

[c] Rg, symbiotically regressive state; STE, Siamese-twins effect; MA, maladjustment; DW, marked withdrawal state; Dep, depression; BID, body image disturbance; ANX, marked anxiety and hypochondriasis; HY, conversion hysteria; Damo, Damocles syndrome; M, hypomania; X, threw the drug away to avoid its side effects.

[d] APD, avoidant personality disorder; DPD, dependent personality disorder; BPD, borderline personality disorder.

[e] HD, hemodialysis; D, dead.

After Four Years

There were 30 surviving patients at 4 years. Even though immunosuppressive drugs have been improved, after 4 years in this study the survival rate of the grafts began to fall below 70%. Therefore most of the recipients who had experienced renal rejection, even if it was mild, were easy prey to the Damocles syndrome [8].

Recipients who died within four years had suffered significantly more frequent psychiatric problems (76.9%) than those who survived. Depression was observed in two recipients over 18 years of age after severe rejection. They suffered from feelings of failure, guilt, and shame; and they considered suicide, with the dilemma of "to be or not to be." Their depressions were more severe than they had been at the 3-year evaluation.

Two subjects were markedly dependent and displayed social withdrawal after recovery from a severe rejection episode. They had been allowed by their mother donors to be excessively dependent or symbiotic. They seemed mildly depressed when they were alone and had fallen into depression after removal of the graft. Four recipients (13.3%) were markedly anxious and had suffered hypochondriasis, remaining in that state since the 3-year evaluation. The other 12 recipients suffered from Damocles syndrome. Conversion hysteria was seen in one boy, who missed his mother's voice after his younger brother entered university, when the mother's attention and expectations appeared to become focused on the brother.

Marked body image disturbance was observed in eight recipients (26.7%: three boys, five girls). Three of them had cenesthopathy of the skin and operation scars; one exhibited psychological rejection of the graft. Four of these subjects threw away the steroid medications to avoid their side effects, two of whom then experienced failure of their graft. The other two recipients suffered from a cushingoid appearance after entrance to high school.

A sexual identity disorder was observed in only one boy, who exhibited this problem soon after transplantation. Other identity disorders were observed in eight recipients, all older than 14 years. They were confused not only by their social identity but also by their self-identity and body image. Six of the eight were on a progressively worsening course from their transplant and were being strictly controlled by their parents. The other two were having a good recovery.

Personality disorder was observed in 10 subjects (33.3%) after graduation from high school; 55.8% of this group were older than 19 years. Although their transplant was doing well, seven exhibited avoidance behavior; the two whose transplants were deteriorating had dependent personality disorders. Borderline personality disorder with acting-out was observed in one girl on a physically excellent course.

Discussion

When we discuss psychiatric problems associated with kidney transplantation, we must not neglect the fact that Japanese hemodialysis treatment has attained the highest level of sophistication in the world. Some patients and their families consider that hemodialysis is safer, more effective, and more inexpensive than kidney transplantation if familial and social supports are available. Therefore the plight of children with renal failure and their mothers' fear of death are not as serious as during the early days when kidney transplantation was the last resort, and if it failed one returned to hemodialysis. Hence kidney transplants are not as widely performed as might be expected. Only about 3% of possible transplant recipients who are on dialysis undergo transplantation and want the organ to be from a living donor (close relative); about 10% of the patients register to receive a transplant from a cadaveric donor. In fact, some patients have refused transplantation even when given this precious chance.

Problems of Donor Selection

In adult cases, donor selection has not necessarily gone smoothly, with donor candidates camouflaging their motives [7, 9, 10]. In the early cases, the donor's decision was frequently influenced by the doctor's or recipient's demands and became an emotional reaction to the recipient's suffering. In fact, most of the organ donations for children were based on an emotional reaction to the recipient's suffering and grief [6]. During most of the decision-making process, *giri* (duty, as a responsibility to the other person's confidence in her or him, or a sense of decency), the duty and responsibility as a parent (or to meet a debt to the recipient's family), and *sekentei* (paying attention to what close relatives think) played the main roles. Particularly, the motivations of sibling donors were complex, and some of them had an actual debt to repay. Sometimes the "black sheep" of the family was selected as donor by ostracism or by pressure for reinstatement into the family [7, 9–11]. There frequently were secret dealings between the chief member of the family and the donor candidates [7, 9]. Hence many of the recipients who had unsolved problems concerning the donor selected tended to suffer from psychiatric problems after transplantation, when they realized that these problems existed (or that the graft was failing).

Donor selection went more smoothly for young recipients than in the adult cases. Most parent donors had made the decision to donate their kidney soon after the child had started on dialysis; troubles at school and worries about entrance to high school enhanced their decision. The most telling influences on acceptance of the procedure came from newspaper stories and television programs.

Most of the mother donors said they would give their child everything they could to help him or her, and they seemed to make the decision to donate a kidney without hesitation. In fact, however, their decisions were emotional reactions to their children, and most of the mothers were seeking rational reasons to justify their consent from close relatives, particularly mothers-in-law and husbands, before their decision. These relatives actually spent a great deal of time persuading them to donate.

We considered it a problem that there were differences between the motivation expressed at the first interview and the real intention that came to light after transplantation. Most of these real intentions leaked out as messages of encouragement and were revealed at interviews during the hospitalization. When the real intention was exposed, the adolescent subjects felt it as a heavy burden and felt a need to respond to the parent's expectations; the young recipient was loaded with guilt. However, the subjects were so dependent on their mothers that their hostilities were accepted by the mothers, and the adolescents were forced into excessive adjustment [2]. The situation was compounded when they became maladjusted or when the donated kidney was rejected; they then felt further guilt and tended to develop psychiatric problems.

The other problem was that the mother donors were eager to welcome the "rebirth" of the subject after transplantation and the release from dialysis. They did not, however, necessarily consider their other children's sacrifices. Some of the recipient's siblings therefore suffered from school avoidance, psychosomatic problems, or delinquency when they were not paid more attention by the mother even after the subject was in good health.

In contrast to the mothers, the father donors, who were not as willing to donate a kidney, not only felt relief for the subject but were relieved that the family as a whole could regain a healthy life. Another problem with father donors was that, unlike the mothers and some of the mother donors, whose real intention was to be free from care of the subject, the mothers did not understand the therapy adequately and missed some of the problems having to do with that therapy, such as the child's throwing the drugs away or signs of rejection or complications.

Psychiatric Problems Just Before Transplantation

As previously described, overprotective mothers encouraged the child's regressive state and selfish behavior. Overanxious mothers were excessively safety-conscious and interfered in the recipient's life, resulting in the child's becoming reclusive and nervous. Both types of mothers thus interfered with the process of separation-individuation of the recipients. The children over 10 years of age were conscious that their physical strength and scholastic ability were less than that of their peers. This situation was also shown by the Rorschach test, as reported by Bouras et al. [12].

Because of the intensive hemodialysis required, the subject under 12 years of age believed that transplantation could bring not only relief from dialysis but also good health. None of the subjects over 13 years old considered their long-term prognosis, immediate death, nor future development.

Among those under 15 years of age before transplantation, none exhibited a delirious state, marked withdrawal, nor depression. We did find that many of the children were regressive and had established a symbiotic relationship with their mothers.

Psychiatric Problems After Living Kidney Transplantation

With living donor kidney transplantation, the donation represents the donor's sacrifice; to carry this idea further, recipients are sometimes given not only a donor's kidney but also the donor's affection, expectations, and sometimes hatred. Recipients' psychological responses to donors are so complex that renal rejection induces in the recipient fear of rejection by their living donor. Most of the psychiatric problems reported for adult recipients are closely related not only to fear of renal rejection and death but also to a guilt-shame feeling toward the donor and fear that the donor and the recipients' relatives may be lost [9–11, 13, 14]. In other words, the most important task for the Japanese recipient of a living kidney from a close relative is to conquer a sense of guilt-shame that is felt toward the donor [2, 6].

In our young subjects almost all the psychiatric problems derived from the donor-recipient relationship. According to their development, however, these problems gradually resembled those of adults, especially after the young person had graduated from high school. Compared with the adults, the adolescent recipients suffered more readily from a lack of self-esteem, disturbed body image, and uncertain identity. Many of them were not enjoying their new lives, which were now relieved from hemodialysis. This lack of enjoyment was due to the fact that they had had short healthy lives prior to transplantation and no experience of dealing with social situations.

Table 3. Psychiatric problems after transplantation (within 3 years).

Psychiatric problem	Subject ($n = 32$)		Adult ($n = 147$)	
Delirious	0		17	11.6%
Manic	1		5	3.4%
Depression	3	9.4%	45	30.6%
Dependence/withdrawal	3	9.4%	—	—
Overanxious	4	12.5%	30	20.4%
Hysterical symptoms	1		4	2.7%
Maladjustment	3	9.4%	7	4.8%
Regressive/symbiosis	14	43.8%	13	8.8%
Identity disorder	1		4	2.7%
Sexual identity disorder	1		3	2.0%
Body image disorder	5	15.6%	6	4.1%
Total	36 (21 cases), 65.6%		133 (89 cases), 60.5%	

The incidence of psychiatric problems that appeared within 3 years of the surgery was 65.6% (21/32) (Table 3); and if the symbiotic relationship with the mother and the regressive state were excluded, the incidence was 46.8% (15/32). The incidence was higher than that reported by Bernstein [14] (12.5%, seen within 6 months) and similar to that reported by Poznanski et al. [15] (50%, seen within 3 years).

Except for the symbiotic relationship and the regressive state, most of these problems seen within 3 years were precipitated by rejection of the graft. All recipients of transplants that were deemed unsuccessful within 2 years (41.7%) showed some problems—in marked contrast to the others subjects.

After 4 years the survival rate of the graft began to decrease. The incidence of graft survival was 62% (71.4% among the unsuccessful transplants, 50% among the surviving transplants, and none of the transplants whose results were excellent and do not undergo rejection). The incidence was lower than that reported by Poznanski et al. [15] (70%, seen after 4–10 years) or by Khan et al. [16] (85.7% seen within 5 years).

The incidence of subjects who experienced renal rejection, even if mild, was markedly higher than that in other studies. In Japan, a good recovery course after transplantation is considered to justify the appearance of psychiatric and other problems [3].

Symbiotic Regressive State

The symbiotic regressive state was the most characteristic problem soon after transplantation. It was observed in 14 children (43.8%) and in 58.3% of the mother donors. If we include mild and brief cases, the incidence reached 60%.

Muslin [8] discussed a similar state, suggested by alimentary symbiosis. There are few reports of this problem from the United States and Europe, except in infantile recipients. We considered that this state was similar to regressively dependent attachment [13], passive dependency [16], and bizarre relations between donor and recipient [17].

The high incidence of this state is thought to be related to the close, mutually bound relationship between the Japanese mother and child. This situation has interfered with the separation-individuation process [18]. A feeling of union, a sense of having achieved the impossible, and a rebirth fantasy interferes with the separation-individuation process and mental development, creating excessive dependency.

When mothers protect their child excessively, it prolongs the child's problem of coping with real-life situations. In contrast to recipients of kidneys from mother donors, we did not observe this state in the recipients of organs from father donors, except in one case, whose problem was reversed more rapidly than in the others.

These affected recipients were prevented from confronting real life and so were protected from severe psychiatric problems. However, the state delayed their mental development and it was only during the latter half of adolescence that their unsolved problems emerged. As many authors [12, 14, 16, 19] have predicted would occur, these five children showed no abnormalities on the Rorschach test or on the Wechsler Intelligence Scale for Children—Revised (WISC-R).

Depression, Marked Dependence, Withdrawal

In adult transplant recipients the most serious psychiatric problem has been depression (incidence 19%–32%) [15, 20–22]. Depression was observed in adult recipients in whom the transplant was unsuccessful within 1 year, who were not as well as they had expected to be because of repeated graft rejections or complications, or who were discouraged by removal of the graft. Most depressions were also related to high-dosage steroids [10, 13, 14, 16, 17].

In our young subjects, depression was observed in six recipients (18.8%) after graft failure. All were more than 14 years of age. This incidence was similar to that for major depression (21.4%) reported by Khan et al. [16] but lower than that for moderate and severe depression (33.3%) reported by Poznanski et al. [15].

Depression that occurred within 3 years of follow-up was observed in three subjects, two of whom were reacting to unsuccessful results that occurred within 2 months of the transplant.

After 4 years, depression was observed in two 18-year-old subjects after anticipation of graft removal. They were suffering severe depressions, pessimism, a guilt-shame feeling toward the donor, loss of a reason for living, and ideas of suicide over the dilemma "to be or not to be," similar to the dilemma "fear of death and fear of life," as reported by Beard [13]. These two young people seemed too tired of living to comply with expectations or investigations of the donor and close relatives. They had graduated from high school, realized the difficulty they had living socially, and wondered if they had anything to live for.

Marked dependence and withdrawal were observed in six recipients. They had no severe trouble at school, but at home they were excessively dependent on the mother donors and derived no pleasure from and had no interest in their surroundings. Especially when they were alone, they seemed to be dysphoric or slightly depressed. This state resembled adolescent depression, but their moods and symptoms (insomnia, anorexia, guilt-shame) were changeable depending on their situations; they and their relatives did not feel depressed. However, three of them over 16 years of age fell into depression after they realized they had lost the graft (the donor's gift) and perhaps their future (Table 4). We considered that the state was similar to those states described as pronounced withdrawn depression [6], some depression [15], social withdrawal [14], excessive dependency and depression, or regressive symptoms [20].

Generally, major depression was observed in adolescents over 13 years of age in Japan. Depression was observed in subjects over 16 years of age. The same situations did not necessarily induce depression in subjects below age 13 years. Poznanski et al.

Table 4. Psychiatric problems after transplantation
(after 4 years).

Psychiatric problem	Subject ($n = 30$)	
Delirious	0	
Manic	0	
Depression	3	(10.0%)
Dependence/withdrawal	3	(10.0%)
Overanxious	4	(13.3%)
Hysterical symptoms	1	
Maladjustment	7	(23.3%)
Regressive/symbiosis	2	
Identity disorder	8	(26.7%)
Sexual identity disorder	1	
Body image disorder	8	(26.7%)
Personality disorder	10	(33.3%)
Total	47 (18 cases), 60.0%	

[15] also reported that moderate and severe depressions were found only in subjects who were older than 15 years.

Possible reasons why depression was not observed in subjects below 15 years of age are as follows.

1. The subject was allowed to depend on the donor excessively, so he or she did not suffer the loss, grief, self-punishment, or the guilt-shame feeling, which were important factors disposing toward depression [23].
2. The subject could not describe his or her inner experiences or feelings accurately, so the relatives did not notice any changes or had thought the state to be a natural reaction to renal rejection. The recipient's feelings and behavior seemed transient and changed according to the situation.
3. The subject did not waste mental energy trying to escape from the state because he or she did not feel mentally ill.

In other words, when the subjects were able to realize that the loss of the graft (or gift) was the loss of *amae* (positive object love) and began to fear punishment or guilt-shame toward their donors, they fell into depression. We believe that the guilt-shame feeling, self-punishment, and loss of *amae* are the factors that are most important and most closely related to depression, stimulating the lowering of self-esteem and causing useless exhaustion of mental energy to regain self-esteem or *amae*.

Marked Anxiety, Hypochondriasis, Conversion Hysteria

Markedly neurotic states (anxiety, hypochondriasis, conversion hysteria) were observed in 12 of our subjects. Except for conversion hysteria, however, these states were observed only when the subjects were in the hospital for treatment of renal rejection or complications. They were not as anxious in their homes, although anxiety was induced by their mother donors, who themselves were markedly anxious and feared graft rejection or death of their child.

After the subjects were finally forced to be independent by their mother donors, they experienced separation anxiety or fear of abandonment, and some of them fell prey to Damocles syndrome [8]. Graduation from middle school or entrance to high school was the most frequent crisis; it separated them from friends who had been supportive since the beginning of dialysis and exposed them to new school fellows (because of the Japanese education system) with whom they had difficulty communicating. These situations led them to avoid or withdraw from social life, or to establish a limited one. Some of them therefore tended to become highly hypochondriacal.

Conversion hysteria was observed in two subjects who had had the full attention of close relatives. When they lost the center position in their family because of their successful transplant or felt fear of abandonment, they fell into hysteria. One girl was afraid of losing the love of her mother donor after severe renal rejections, and one boy had difficulty tolerating the sound of his mother donor's voice after his father died and his younger brother succeeded in university; he (the subject) realized then that he had lost his leading role in the family.

Delirious State

The delirious state was not observed in any of the subjects despite the high dosage of steroids required. Delirium had been observed in 7.0% of the adult recipients of living donor kidneys and in 26.9% of the adult recipients of cadaveric kidneys. The delirium in adults was closely related to the high dosage of steroids and the discouragement those adults felt after the failed treatment for graft rejection. We believe that the delirious state was induced not only by the steroids but also by other factors, such as arteriosclerosis, physical dysfunction, and discouragement or collapse.

Body Image Disturbance, Identity Disorders, Personality Disorders

The evaluations of the recipients by their parents were more lenient than those reported in the United States and Europe [9, 19, 23, 24]. The male recipients seemed to be adjusted superficially and were considered by their parents to be more obedient and less dependent than the female recipients. In fact, however, they tended to be over-attentive and doted on their parents to compensate for the parent's sacrifices and gift; they often demonstrated hostile dependency. The female recipients suffered from distortion of body image and became alexithimic and retiring in school, though they were thought to be less dependent and less regressive by their parents. The girls felt less guilt but were more dependent than the boys. The differences were believed due to boys' heavier burden to meet their donor's expectations and the more burdensome social expectation for boys. This result was similar to that when we studied the social image of adult hemodialysis patients [5].

Body Image Disturbance

We observed 10 recipients (four boys, six girls) who were suffering excessively from the cushingmoid appearance, strange sensations on the skin, or surgical scars. Five adolescent subjects were having difficulty integrating the grafts into their body image [7, 24]. The first set of problems (personal appearance) became more serious after entrance to high school. The latter problem was related to their relationship with the donor. Three of the latter subjects demonstrated a Siamese-twins effect [7] within 3 years along with a symbiotic relationship. Two boys with father donors showed a psychological rejection of the grafts, as the responsibility of meeting their father's expectations for their social adjustment became too heavy.

Body image disturbances among these young people were so serious that they were unable to enjoy their new life; the problem was related to a lack of communication with their new school fellows. Only five of them, who had had many friends before transplantation, improved their adjustment significantly after transplantation. Their physical status was really too serious for them to secretly throw out their steroid medications, as reported by Korsch et al. [17]. Nevertheless, two of the kidney recipients caused the grafts to be rejected by throwing out the drugs.

Integration of the grafts into their body image progressed more smoothly than in the adults, who suffered from heavy feelings of obligation and guilt-shame toward their donors and close relatives. In contrast with the adults, most of the young subjects did not talk about the transplanted kidney, except when the transplant was the topic under discussion. Their integration was superficial, however, and most of them began to suffer from body image disturbances after they were required to be independent. Two of them showed psychological rejection of their father's kidney after they failed to adjust socially in the way their father donor had hoped.

Three recipients who were in a symbiotic relationship with their mother donors showed the Siamese-twins effect [7] after rejection. They were early subjects whose transplants were done against their father's will (two of the fathers were physicians); both they and their mother donors had extreme fear of rejection.

Identity Disorder

Eight recipients suffered from social identity and self-identity disturbances. They found it difficult to use common sense with their new school fellows and to enjoy their donated but limited new lives. Most of their self-images or their body images were not improved, as Korsch et al. [17] and others [25, 26] have pointed out, especially after renal rejection in adolescents. After entrance to high school they began to suffer increasingly from being unable to live like their new school fellows, even when they made very effort to communicate or to identify with their new friends.

In American and European reports [9, 14, 15, 17] the donors kept the recipients at a distance in order to encourage them to be independent. In Japan, almost all the mother continued to shower the subject with love and allowed excessive dependence in order to keep their own peace of mind after transplantation. Moreover, most of the father donors had excessive expectations without providing appropriate support. Therefore the subject and the parent donors were mutually bound, and it was easy for the parents to control the behavior of the child. Some of the subjects began to suffer a loss of self, feeling the control exerted by their parents. They felt it was difficult to meet the parents' wishes or expectations to the extent that two them showed psychological rejection of their donated kidneys.

Sex Identity Disorder

In the United States and Europe sexual disorders are often reported and discussed psychoanalytically [12, 14, 16, 17, 27]. Among our recipients, only one boy, who received a kidney from his mother, had a sexual identity disorder for an extended time after rejection. We presume that this disorder occurs rarely in Japan despite the cross-sexual transplants, because of "maternalism," as we call it.

Personality Disorder

A personality disorder was observed in 10 recipients who were over 18 years of age. Korsch et al. [17] reported that child transplant recipients had lower self-esteem than healthy children and patients with other chronic illnesses, but the incidence of personality disorders in their study and ours are not different between the recipients less than 16 years of age whose grafts survived and those whose grafts did not survive. We did observe personality disorders more frequently in recipients who had a difficult course of recovery even if the grafts survived. These subjects had unsolved problems in their families: two parents had been under hemodialysis, one father had died before transplantation, three parents became more troublesome than before, two fathers had opposed transplantation even afterward, and three patients with early-onset personality disorder (before 6 years of age) had had a symbiotic relationship with the mother and were still mutually bound.

The period before and after graduation from high school was the most critical for the adolescent subjects. After transplantation their personality disorders gradually were revealed by their inability to deal with familiar problems and real life. Two of them exhibited avoidance behavior, seven had a dependent personality disorder, and one girl with an excellent recovery course was revealed to have a borderline personality disorder with acting out (e.g., wrist cutting and violence to her mother after her father's hospitalization and loss of her mother's support).

Conclusion

Many adolescent recipients given transplants of living donor kidneys from a parent suffered various psychiatric problems, as has been reported from the United States [27]. The problems were more related to mutually bound relationships with their mother donor than with their father donor and were due to interference with the separation-individuation process.

The suffering of the adolescent recipients is so serious that ordinary psychotherapy is not necessarily effective and make-shift therapeutic approaches have often been harmful [9, 24, 28, 29]. We have supported these subjects using a long-range plan so they can enjoy their new lives and can develop normally. We provide effective, comprehensive liaison-consultation services not only to these adolescent recipients and their families but also to young patients with renal disease and other chronic illnesses.

References

1. Sato K, Miura S (1977) Psychiatric problems related to the process of living kidney donor selection. In: Koshiba K, Sakai T (eds) Annual report, Kidney Center, Kitasato University Hospital. Part 3 (in Japanese). Kitasato University Hospital, Kidney Center, Sagamihara, Japan, pp 26–43
2. Sato K (1978) Psychiatric problems after kidney transplantation (in Japanese). Psychiatr Neurol Jpn 80:65–83
3. Sato K (1979) Enclosed anger-agression seen through recipient of kidney transplantation. In: Hara T, Shikano T (eds) Aggression from the standpoint of psychiatrists (in Japanese). Iwasaki Academic Press, Tokyo, pp 115–142
4. Sato K, Suzuki Y, Akahoshi K, Miura S (1983) Psychiatric problems of recipients of cadaveric kidney transplantation. In: Miura S (ed) Tenth anniversary selected papers of Kitasato psychiatry

1971–1980. Department of Psychiatry Kitasato University, School of Medicine, Sagamihara, Japan, pp 130–145

5. Sato K, Fukuyama Y, Ziller R, et al (1885) Social-image of hemodialysis patients—through self-other oriented method (in Japanese). Jpn J Clin Dialysis 1:1095–1105

6. Sato K, Akahoshi K, Suzuki Y, Miura S, et al (1990) Psychiatric problems of children and adolescents who had living kidney transplantation (in Japanese). Jpn J Child Adolesc Psychiatry 31:327–350

7. Muslin HL (1971) On acquiring a kidney. Am J Psychiatry 127:1185–1188

8. Koocher GP, O'Malley JE (1981) The Damocles syndrome. McGraw-Hill, New York

9. Kemph JP, Bermann EA, Capolillo HP (1969) Kidney transplant and shifts in family dynamics Am J Psychiatry 125:1485–1490

10. Abram HS, Buchanann DC (1977) The gift of life; a review of the psychological aspects of kidney transplantation. Int J Psychiatr Med 7:153–164

11. Cramond WA (1978) Renal transplantation—experiences with recipients and donors. In: Castelnuovo-Tedesco P (ed) Psychiatric aspects of transplantation. Grune & Stratton, Orlands, pp 116–132

12. Bouras M, Silverstre D, Broyer D, Reinbault G (1976) Renal transplantation in children; a psychological survey, Clin Nephrol 6:478–482

13. Beard BH (1969) Fear of death and fear of life; the dilemma in chronic renal failure, hemodialysis and kidney transplantation. Arch Gen Psychiatry 21:1189–1193

14. Bernstein NM (1971) After transplantation—the child's emotional reactions. Am J Psychiatry 127:1189–1193

15. Poznanski EO, Miller E, SalGuero C, Keich RC (1978) Quality of life for long-term survivors of end-stage renal disease. JAMA 239:2443–2447

16. Kahn AU, Herdon CH, Ahmadian HP (1973) Social and emotional adaptations of children with transplanted kidneys and hemodialysis. Am J Psychiatry 127:1194–1198

17. Korsch BM, negrete VF, Fine RN, et al (1973) Kidney transplantation in children: psychosocial follow-up study on child and family. J Pediatr 83:399–408

18. Starkman MB (1980) Psychological problems resulting from parent-to-adolescent renal transplantation. Gen Hosp Psychiatry 2:289–293

19. Crittenden MA, Holliday MA, Piel CF, et al (1985) Intellectual development of children with renal insufficiency and end stage. Int J Pediatr Nephrol 6:275–280

20. Ferris GN (1969) Psychiatric considerations in patients receiving cadaveric renal transplantation. South Med J 62:1482–1484

21. Frank G (1974) Psychopathologish Befund vor und nach Nieren Transplantation. Fortschr Neurol Psychiatr 42:156–162

22. Wilson WP, Stickel DL, Hayes CP, et al (1968) Psychiatric considerations of renal transplantation. Arch Intern Med 122:502–506

23. Bemporad J (1987) Manifest symptomatology and psychodynamics of depression in childhood and adolescents. In: Arieti S, Bemporad J (eds) Severe and mild depression. Basic Books, New York

24. Kaplan De-Nour A (1979) Adolescents adjustment to chronic hemodialysis. Am J Psychiatry 36:430–433

25. Fine RN, Malekzadeh MH, Korsch BM, et al (1978) Longterm results of renal transplantation in children. Pediatrics 61:641–650

26. Basch S (1973) The intra-psychic integration of new organ: a clinical study of kidney transplantation. Psychoanal Q 42:364–384

27. Zarinski I (1975) Psychological problems of kidney transplanted adolescents. Adolescence 10:101–107

28. Sampson TF (1975) The child in renal failure: emotional impact of treatment on the child and his family. J Am Acad Child Psychiatry 14:462–476

29. Drotar D (1975) The treatment of a severe anxiety reaction in adolescent boy following kidney transplantation. J Am Acad Child Psychiatry 14:451–461

Child Abuse and Parental Power in Japan

Shinichiro Kado[1] and Kotaro Nakayama[2]

Summary. We reviewed four nationwide studies on child abuse in Japan done in 1973, 1983, 1984, and 1988. It is difficult to draw any conclusion about the trend of child abuse from these studies because the definitions of abuse were not the same. However, we can find no evidence to show an increase of child abuse in Japan, although it is not difficult to imagine that hidden cases overwhelmingly outnumber the reported cases. We estimate the provisional incidence at 45.8 per 1000 children in Japan. Regarding child abuse cases, in general, legal intervention is believed to be ineffective in Japan, although its effectiveness is indicated in the findings of the research done by the Directors of the Child Guidance Centers in 1988. We believe that the Child Guidance Centers should not be reluctant to use judicial power to protect the human rights of a child.

Key words. Child abuse—Incidence—Parental power—Forfeiture

It has been said that the incidence of child abuse is low in Japan. However, many of those concerned have recently pointed out that a large number of child abuse cases, especially sexual ones, are kept secret by family members and are not reported by neighbors, doctors, or teachers [1]. Although we have no firm data of the incidence of child abuse in Japan, UNICEF [2] has been concerned about infant abuse in the world, citing recent statistics (Table 1). At the moment, internationally comparable statistics are available only for infants under 1 year of age, although most abused children are not infants but children of the age range 2–4 years. From the data in Table 1, we cannot but infer that the incidence of other varieties of child abuse in Japan must be underestimated. Here we review the results of the nationwide studies on child abuse, examining the annual number of cases and some problems arising in the management of child abuse cases.

[1] Kyoto City Child Welfare Center, Takeyamachi-Sembon-Higashi, Kamigyo-ku, Kyoto 602, Japan
[2] Department of Neuropsychiatry, Faculty of Medicine, Kyoto University, Shogoin-Kawaharacho, Sakyo-ku, Kyoto 606, Japan

Table 1. Death of infants from presumed abuse, 1985–1990.

Country	Deaths/100 000 live births
Former Czechoslovakia	10.1
United States	9.8
Former Soviet Union	8.7
Denmark	8.1
Japan	7.4
New Zealand	6.9
Finland	6.2
Hungary	5.7
Australia	5.5
Switzerland	4.9
Bulgaria	4.3
Austria	4.3
Belgium	4.3
United Kingdom	3.9
Germany	3.5
France	3.1
Canada	2.7
Poland	2.4
The Netherlands	2.1
Norway	1.7
Sweden	0.9
Italy	0.4
Spain	0.2

Reported and Unreported Cases

So far, four nationwide studies on child abuse have been conducted in Japan. It was around the time of the second baby-boom, from 1971 to 1973, that child abuse became a national concern in Japan for the first time. During those years "coin-locker babies' were often reported in the media (infants who were killed or simply abandoned in coin-operated lockers in big railway stations). This was just after the end of the income-doubling policy from 1960 to 1970, which was accompanied by rapid urbanization of the whole country. This miserable phenomenon was considered serious pathology emerging in a rapidly developing society. It was argued that the main cause of this pathology was the loss or decline of the capacity of child rearing in urban families.

1973 Study

The Ministry of Health [3] carried out the first nationwide study on child abuse during the period from 1 April 1973 to 31 March 1974 using a questionnaire to be filled out by the directors of all the child guidance centers ($n = 153$). They were asked to report the numbers of killed, almost lethally abused, and deserted children under age 3 years. The numbers of these categories were 236, 36, and 139, respectively, giving a total of only 411.

1983 Study

Ten years later another study was carried out. It was a 1-year investigation by a nongovernmental group of experts called the Research Group on Child Abuse [4]

Table 2. One-year investigation by the Research Group on Child Abuse: April 1983 to March 1984.

Type of abuse	No.
Physical abuse	223
Sexual abuse	46
Subtotal	*269*
Emotional abuse	34
Neglect or refusal of custody	111
Others	2
Total	416

Table 3. One-month investigation by the Association of Directors of Child Guidance Centers: February 1984.

Parameter	No. of cases, February 1984	Estimated annual number[a]	
		A	B
Abuse	67 (4.2%)	1222	804
Desertion	30 (1.9%)	553	360
Total	97 (6.1%)	1775	1164

[a] A, Based on February 1984 figures; B, based on monthly figures.

(Table 2). From 1 April 1983 to 31 March 1984, Ikeda and her colleagues received 416 reports of child abuse from the directors of all the child guidance centers ($n = 164$). They defined child abuse in a stricter way than in the previous study, that is, as "intrafamilial child abuse by parents or other custodians."

1984 Study

Another 1-month study was conducted by the Association of Directors of Child Guidance Centers [5] in which they investigated only two categories: abuse and desertion (Table 3). The total number of all clients in February 1984 was 1581, and during the fiscal year 1983 the number was 29103. Based on the rates of the two categories, the estimated annual numbers for child abuse and desertion were 1222 and 553, respectively. They also estimated the annual numbers of 804 and 360, respectively, based on the monthly numbers multiplied by 12.

1988 Study

The Association of Directors of Child Guidance Centers, mentioned above, conducted a second investigation from 1 April 1988 to 30 September of 1988 (6 months). With the purpose of conducting study relative to the 1983 research reported by the Research Group, they studied four categories using the same definitions as those of the former research group [5] and added parents' prohibiting their child from going to school, bullying and other types of abuse, and neglect. The rate of response was 100%. The results and the estimated annual numbers are shown in Table 4. Based on the results of this study, it was estimated that the rate of child abuse by parents or

Table 4. Six-month investigation by the Association of Directors of Child Guidance Centers: April to September 1988.

Parameter	Cases	×2 (Annual)
Physical abuse	275	550
Sexual abuse	48	96
Subtotal	*323*	*646*
Emotional abuse	68	136
Neglect or refusal of custody	391	782
Desertion	229	458
Prohibited from going to school	28	56
Total	1039	2078

other custodians is 0.066 per 1000 children. In urban areas (Tokyo and 10 other designated large cities) the rate is higher than in rural areas (0.098 versus 0.059 per 1000).

Trend of Child Abuse in Japan

It is difficult to draw any conclusions about the trend of child abuse from the studies in 1973, 1983, 1984, and 1988 because the definitions of abuse varied. For example, in the 1973 study the researchers dealt only with lethal abuse of children under age 3. It might be possible to compare the results of the 1983, 1984, and 1988 studies because these three studies included common categories. When we estimate the annual amount of abuse in a narrow sense (physical and sexual abuse together) during the fiscal year 1983, we may get the following three different numbers depending on the means of estimation: 269 cases, 1222 cases, or 804 cases (Tables 2, 3). It is unreasonable to compare these different estimations with that of 1988 (646 cases) (Table 4).

Kamiide [6] also reasonably described the difficulty of the time series study of their two investigations (the 1984 and 1988 studies). He argued that the former dealt only with desertion and physical and sexual abuse. He estimated the total annual number of these three categories in the 1984 study as 1164. This figure exceeded the number in the 1988 study of 1104 (458 + 550 + 96) (Table 4). He stated that it was difficult to conclude directly from these investigations that child abuse is markedly increasing in Japan. On the other hand, Ikeda, some other authors, and the Federation of Japanese Bar Associations suggested that there is an increase in child abuse in Japan. We agree with Kamiide's conclusion that there is no evidence to indicate an increase in child abuse in Japan.

It is not difficult to imagine, however, that hidden cases overwhelmingly outnumber the reported cases in the 1988 study. In 1986 in England and Wales, 2137 cases were registered as child abuse and neglect, with a rate of 2.29 per 1000 children. However, the actual number of abuse cases in England and Wales was thought to be 10 times as many as the number of registered cases [7]. Again, according to the data cited by UNICEF (Table 1), the rate of infant deaths due to presumed abuse in Japan is twice as high as in the United Kingdom. Therefore the actual prevalence of child abuse in Japan may well be at least 20 times that of the reported rate of registered cases in England and Wales. Thus we could provisionally estimate the prevalence of child abuse and neglect in Japan at 45.8 per 1000 children.

Few cases of child abuse (especially sexual abuse) are reported to the Child Guidance Centers in Japan. It is partly because the system of reporting does not function well. According to the Child Welfare Act, whoever finds or suspects child abuse or neglect is obliged to report it to a child guidance center. Unlike European countries and the United States, we have no statute defining who may report the case without likelihood of legal reprisal, and who must report under threat of civil or criminal penalty. This uncertainty is one of the main reasons we have such a small number of reported cases in Japan.

Parental Power in Japan

Historically, the motto "rich country and strong military," which has applied since the Meiji Restoration (1868) was associated with the feudal patriarchal family system called "Ie" (which literally means "house"), where a patriarch was required to be responsible for all family affairs. With some assistance of the parens patrie power, the patriarch was permitted to do whatever he wanted to all members of his Ie. After surrender to the United Nations' military force, the penal and civil codes were only partly amended according to the standards of the Western countries at that time. Nevertheless, parental power has remained strong. It tends to be interpreted as power and authority rather than responsibility and duty.

In the Japanese Civil Code (Act 89, 1896; partly amended in 1949) and the Mental Health Act (Act 123, 1950), parental power comprises the following elements:

1. The right and the duty of having custody of the child, educating the child (CC s. 820), and consenting to compulsory psychiatric hospitalization (Mental Health Act s. 33)
2. The duty of paying for any damage the child or the mentally ill person under a parent's supervision has caused to a third person (CC ss. 709 and 714)
3. The right of designating the place of residence of the child (CC s. 821)
4. The right of personally chastizing the child or of placing it in a disciplinary institution with the permission of the Family Court (CC s. 822)
5. The right of giving permission to carry on an occupation (CC s. 823)
6. The right to give permission for marriage of a minor child (CC s. 737)
7. The duty of managing the property of a child and of representing the child on judicial acts concerning his or her property (CC s. 824)

In the above 1988 study, the Association of the Directors of the Child Guidance Centers mentioned that the strong parental power in Japan was the most serious difficulty when dealing with child abuse, and that 113 cases of parental refusal to have their abused children removed to a children's home were reported over a 6-month period. It occurred because usual placement in a children's home is a kind of commission contract between a guardian or a person with parental power and a children's home, which is under the Child Welfare Act (Act 164, 1947), Section 27. Therefore when the guardian or person with parental power opposes the placement, the child guidance center cannot carry it out. It is understood that this opposition is based on the right and duty of having custody of and educating the child (CC s. 820) and the right of designation the place of residence of the child (CC s. 821).

Table 5. Number of applications and approvals regarding Section 28.

Parameter	'82	'83	'84	'85	'86	'87	'88	'89	'90	'91
Applications	6	4	14	3	0	5	6	3	19	10
Approvals	3	4	13	3	1	5	3	0	15	9

Data from the Ministry of Health and Welfare, 1982–1992 [8].

Partial Forfeiture of Parental Power

The Child Welfare Act, Section 28, sets forth the measures that the governor of the prefecture is to take in case of abuse or serious neglect of a child. In this section, it is stated that when a parent or other custodian abuses a child or seriously neglects its custody, thereby leading to serious infringement of the child's welfare, the child can be removed from the custodian's custody; and if the guardian or person with parental power opposes placement of the child in a children's home, the governor of the prefecture may order such placement without the custodian's agreement under a ruling of the Family Court. It is said there is no regulation regarding partial forfeiture of parental power in the Japanese laws, but this Section 28 could be regarded as partial, temporary forfeiture of parental power.

Nevertheless, directors of children's homes complain that even in case of placement by the governor, they could not stop the child's discharge against the objections of parents or custodians. Therefore they consider Section 28 to be ineffective. Such an unhappy situation might well occur because there is no provision setting forth that the Family Court shall hear a child in question and investigate circumstances before the discharge of the child.

The 1988 investigation carried out by the Association of the Directors of the Child Guidance Centers over a 6-month period showed that 20 (3.2%) of the 624 children who had been placed in children's homes under Section 27 had been discharged by parents who used coercion. However, it also reported that none of the six children who had been placed in children's homes under a ruling of the Family Court (under Section 28) had been taken away. Therefore the authors consider that Section 28 must be effective. Unfortunately, child guidance centers seldom use it (Table 5), as they believe that it is not effective. The directors of child guidance centers should reconsider Section 28; moreover, if the condition of discharge is defined clearly in the Act, the measures under this section should become more effective and more reliable for the directors of children's homes.

Total Forfeiture of Parental Power

The Civil Code, Section 834, sets forth the forfeiture of parental power. This section states that if a father or mother abuses parental power or is guilty of gross misconduct the Family Court may, on application of any of the child's relatives or of a public prosecutor, adjudge the forfeiture of parental power. Section 835 sets forth forfeiture of the power of managing property. However, there is no provision for forfeiture of any other part of parental power, although Section 28 of the Child Welfare Act can provide partial forfeiture, as mentioned above.

Abuse or neglect is committed mostly in families isolated from their relatives; the spouse of an abuser is often an accomplice in the maltreatment, and the siblings are

Table 6. Number of applications and approvals regarding Section 834.

Parameter	'82	'83	'84	'85	'86	'87	'88	'89	'90	'91
Applications	3	0	2	1	0	0	1	0	2	2
Approvals	2	1	0	0	1	0	0	0	0	3

Data from the Ministry of Health and Welfare, 1982–1992 [8].

also victims and have no access to a public prosecutor. Thus Section 33-5 of the Child Welfare Act prescribes that a director of a child guidance center can be an applicant for the forfeiture.

Nevertheless, child guidance centers are reluctant to request the forfeiture of parental power to the Family Court. This reluctance is partly because the Japanese prefer an extrajudicial solution to a judicial one and partly because parental power is emphasized more than parental responsibility and duty. In addition, strange to say, a number of directors of child guidance centers believe that the forfeiture of parental power is difficult and has been adjudged only once so far, although it is not true (Table 6). If such a myth made the directors refrain from applying to the Court for the forfeiture, it would be unfortunate for abused children.

Conclusion

In Japan economic development and urbanization appear to have undermined the capabilities of families regarding custody and education. It is reasonable to infer that there must be many more unreported child abuse and neglect cases than are reported. If the report system is improved, the national concern about child abuse and neglect could increase. Moreover, it is desirable that the concept of parental authority should be amended in the penal and civil codes and in other related laws in the direction of the UN Convention of the Rights of the Child, which Japan ratified in 1994.

References

1. Osaka Study Group for Child Abuse (1989) The report of the investigation of the care for abused children (in Japanese). OSGCA, Osaka
2. UNICEF (1994) The progress of nations. UNICEF, New York
3. Ministry of Health and Welfare (1975) Report on cases of child abuse, desertion and killing (in Japanese). MHW, Tokyo
4. Ikeda Y, Tamura K, Shimohira Y, Yoshizawa H (1985) Child abuse (in Japanese). Research Group on Child Abuse, Tokyo
5. Ikeda Y (1987) Child abuse (in Japanese). Chuokoronsha, Tokyo
6. Kamiide H (1989) The summary report by the Chairman of the Association of Child Guidance Center Managers (in Japanese). In: Documentations for the annual meeting of the association, Tokyo
7. Creighton SJ (1987) Annual update of statistics 1986. National Society for the Prevention of Cruelty to Children, London
8. Ministry of Health and Welfare (1982–1992) Annual Report on Social Welfare in Japan (in Japanese). MHW, Tokyo

Training and Education of Child Mental Health Professions in Japan

Kosuke Yamazaki

Summary. In this paper, the status quo of mental health activities in Japan is reviewed from the viewpoint of child and adolescent psychiatry, with particular emphasis on the training of mental health professionals in our country. Multifarious problems constitute the current issues facing child mental health care in Japan, specifically: (1) support for young mothers harboring anxiety with regards to child rearing, (2) psychiatric intervention in the field of school mental health care, particularly with regard to phenomena such as school refusal and bullying, which show no signs of abating, (3) cases of child abuse, especially child sexual abuse, believed to have been a limited phenomenon in Japan, are now surfacing in large numbers, (4) the problem of student apathy related to the system of entrance examinations for colleges and universities in Japan, (5) issues regarding the increasing number of expatriate children returning to Japan, and alternately, issues regarding foreign children entering Japanese schools, arising in proportion to the increase in international exchange, (6) issues arising from the recent rapid progress in medicine, e.g., the effects of artificial insemination and selective birth of male or female offspring on the mental development and character formation of children; various conflicts arising from organ transplantations; the question of dignified life and death seen in terminal care, and (7) issues arising from the increase in nuclear families on the one hand, and multigeneration families living together out of financial necessity on the other hand; the approach to the aging of society; and problems arising from increasing participation of women in the labor force, and the accompanying changes in the mode of child care. The question of how mental health care activities ought to be organized, and how we should go about training the specialists to undertake mental health care in light of these problems—not to mention the mountain of other issues being experienced by mankind for the first time—is reviewed with reference to the history of child and adolescent psychiatry in Japan. Lastly, the state of pre- and postgraduate training in child and adolescent psychiatry being provided by the medical schools in Japan is summarized.

Key words. Training and education in child psychiatry—Child mental health in Japan—Mental health in school children—Japanese culture

Division of Child and Adolescent Psychiatry, Department of Psychiatry and Behavioral Science, Tokai University School of Medicine, Boseidai, Isehara, Kanagawa 259-11, Japan

In comparison to the countries of Europe and the United States, mental health activities in Japan have lagged far behind. The first textbook on modern-day psychiatry used in Japan was the translation of Maudsley's manual translated by Humiya Kanbe in 1876. In 1918, after conducting a survey of psychiatric cases, Shuzou Kure had the following to say about the utterly tragic circumstances surrounding the psychiatric patient in Japan: "The psychiatric patient has, beyond the misfortune of being victim of the disease, the added misfortune of having been born in this country. To help and protect such patients is a matter of ethics, and an issue calling for immediate national attention."

In 1919 legislation regarding psychiatric hospital care was promulgated that incorporated medical doctrine, and various laws regarding mental health care were established. After World War II various systems for mental health care operative in European countries and the United States were incorporated, and it is said that psychiatric care in Japan is now on a par, at least in form, with the care in those countries. However, we are still faced with countless issues yet to be addressed, such as the training of professionals, the maintenance and upgrading of clinical and research facilities (in terms of quality and quantity), and the formulation of clinical teams. It may be true that Japan has undergone rapid economic transformation into an "economic giant" over the last 20 years, but this change has not brought about true affluence perceivable by the public, and perhaps it is this lack in accumulation of social economic wealth that is being reflected in the poverty of mental health activities. It is questionable how far we have been able to redeem or revise the state of mental health care during the half-century since Professor Kure first voiced his distress.

This chapter presents the state of mental health activities in Japan from the standpoint of child and adolescent psychiatry, with special emphasis on the training and education of mental health professionals.

Issues of Mental Health Care for Children in Japan

Several issues have surfaced recently in Japan. First is the problem of anxiety and insecurity in young mothers with regard to raising children. There are increasing numbers of mothers who are wracked with uncertainty until they can seek advice on each and every detail, such as how firm they can be with their children when they are being difficult, or if it is proper to sleep alongside their children in the same bed. Nurturing behavior, which should have been transmitted by tradition or through reading books or learned from their mothers or grandmothers, is perhaps being shaken from its foundations. Hence children are being burdened with an important issue beginning from early infancy: the foundation of human development. Additionally, the trend for parents to seek advice from counseling programs about education and development aired on radio and television is somewhat worrisome. The fact that these people are readily convinced by explanations or advice given in a few minutes is another strange phenomenon. Such a trend highlights the abnormal authority or reliability ascribed to information being transmitted over the mass media—something that needs to be carefully reviewed [1].

The second issue is the problem of school mental health. The incidence of school refusal and bullying in the school continues to rise unabated. The 1990 survey by the Japanese Ministry of Education revealed the largest recorded number (48174) of elementary and junior high school students absent from school for durations of more than 50 days because they disliked school. This figure amounts to 0.34% of the total 14 248 355 elementary and junior high school students in Japan. The figures show that the number of school refusals has risen 2.71-fold among elementary school children and 5.68-fold among junior high students. Recent surveys indicate a tendency of less bullying among schools nationwide, but that the bullying in large cities is not only on the rise but is becoming increasingly treacherous and sinister in nature. The high school enrollment rate is 94.6%, but the dropout rate is showing a gradual increase, amounting to 2.2% in 1990. It is estimated that in Kanagawa Prefecture, where I work at Tokai University, there are more than 20 000 adolescents between 15 and 20 years old who are unable to settle into any school or job. The real problem of school refusal resides in the fact that not going to school has become the strongest card children can play in the face of a society that has prioritized academic qualification to the extreme.

The third issue is child abuse. Various surveys have been conducted in this respect, and increasing numbers of sexual child abuse cases, believed to be uncommon in Japan up to now, and in particular that of girls being abused by their blood-related parents, are being reported. Children who have been abused, who have taken lightly or treated poorly, can be regarded as having problems in common with refugees. It is estimated that there are 15 million refugees worldwide, half of them children. Refugees are defined as people residing outside their mother countries who cannot or will not return to their homeland owing to fear or persecution. There are few psychiatric studies on refugee children, although a survey conducted by the World Psychiatric Association, Child and Adolescent Section, has revealed a high incidence of various disorders among such children. In particular, I was struck by the finding that many of those children have strong feelings of despair with regard to the future. What can we as adults do in this situation in which children in the midst of their development, who ought to be full of hope and dreams, can feel only despair?

Fourth, there are large numbers of college students who spend much of their time in coffee shops. They do what is required of them, but they do not undertake any productive activity on their own. They are said to suffer from "student apathy," although no clear indications of mental disorders can be detected. Many variations exist; one type is the student who gains entry into a first-rate college or university at the first try but who "burns out" the moment he or she enrolls and quickly loses the will to go to school. These students are often perfectionists, lacking flexibility and exhibiting ceremonial behavior. Many of them are quiet, and the parents are apt to comment that their child has always been a well behaved, good child. Many parents regarded scholastic achievement as their only wish regarding their children, and the students with student apathy often state that it was easiest for them to be studying. This phenomenon is related to the college entrance examination system in Japan, wherein gaining entry into a college represents an enormous hurdle; once admitted, however, students are often graduated by an escalator-like process. These students, who have spent their lives focused on their immediate studies with no life plan and who have avoided the social and human aspects of life, lose sight of their goal the moment they enter college [2].

The fifth issue is the problem of expatriate children returning home. Their numbers are increasing in proportion to the promotion of international exchange, as are the numbers of foreign children entering Japanese schools. In addition, many children accompany their fathers in assignments abroad and find it difficult to adjust, experiencing various degrees of culture shock. A researcher from the United States reported on this phenomenon at the Kyoto Congress of the International Association for Child and Adolescent Psychiatry and Allied Professions (IACAPAP). Japanese industry often builds factories abroad, translocates families from Japan, and initiates operations there, taking advantage of the expansive land available, with consideration only for the economic aspects of the venture. In such cases, many junior high and high school students find themselves unable to adjust to the cultural background of the region and come to harbor many psychological problems. They become filled with gloom, isolated from others who understand their culture, and become subject to discrimination in many respects. The converse of this problem is the increasing numbers of elementary and junior high school students who require Japanese-language education who have accompanied their families, who constitute foreign laborers in Japan. At present, there are approximately 5500 foreign children who are unable to speak Japanese but are attending schools in Japan. Many of these children speak Portuguese, Chinese, and Spanish as their first language, and the teachers in Japanese schools are often unable to deal with them. In this day and age of accelerated international exchange, the establishment of concrete methods for resolving such problems is a matter of utmost urgency.

Last, we must touch on child mental health issues arising from the recent rapid advancements in medicine. We are coming face to face with problems never before seen, such as the effects of artificial insemination and the selective birth of male and female offspring on psychological development and character formation, the various emotional conflicts inherent to organ transplantations, and the conflicts regarding dignity of life and death during terminal care. In addition there are issues that arise from changes in society, such as an increase in the number of nuclear families and the co-habitation of multigenerational families due to financial need, the aging of society, the advances of women in society, and the accompanying changes in the practice of bringing up children.

We are faced with a mountain of such problems, both old and new. Mental health activities must address all such wide-ranging issues, not just those regarding mental disorders. In this respect, the specialists cannot remain in their own spheres of specialization. What is required is research and practice of a truly interdisciplinary nature. The issue at hand is how we can educate and train specialists who can stand up to this most important task. The specialties involved with mental health are highly varied, and the following section reports the present state of activities in Japan through a review of the history of child and adolescent psychiatry up to the present.

History of Child and Adolescent Psychiatry in Japan

As early as the early 1900s Shouma Morita, renowned for his Morita therapy, was lecturing on psychosis during childhood. During the 1930s departments of child and adolescent psychiatry were established on a limited scale at the University of Tokyo and the University of Nagoya, where studies were initiated though far removed from the limelight. In 1947 the child welfare law was enacted, and child guidance centers were established in each prefecture of Japan. In 1948 a child psychiatric ward was established at the National Kounodai Hospital, and the first psychiatric hospital for children, the Tokyo Metropolitan Umegaoka Hospital, was opened. During the 1950s the Department of Child Mental Health was established within the National Mental

Health Institute, and more and more cases of infantile autism and school refusal were being reported from universities throughout the country.

It was at about this time that psychiatrists who had studied under such mentors as Drs. Szurek, Bender, Rank, and Kanner started returning to Japan; and in 1958 a Study Group for Child Psychiatry was established within the Japanese Society for Psychiatry and Neurology. Two years later, in 1960, this study group evolved into the Japanese Society of Child and Adolescent Psychiatry (JSCAP).

Child psychiatry, however, has yet to gain official recognition as an independent clinical entity within the Japanese medical system. The operation of child psychiatric wards are burdonsome financially, and there are only 13 such wards throughout Japan at present. All of them are public facilities that qualify for subsidies from the prefecture or city in which they are situated. In 1975 the late Professor Kiyoshi Makita opened a full-time clinic for child and adolescent psychiatry at the Tokai University School of Medicine, but we have yet to see the establishment of child psychiatric departments in any medical school in Japan.

The importance of child psychiatry has come to be appreciated in welfare and educational systems, however, and the 1960s brought with it the establishment of short-term therapeutic institutions as well as special classes for emotionally disturbed children. According to a survey conducted in 1994, there were 4150 special classes for emotionally disturbed children throughout the nation, in which 11 637 elementary and junior high school students were enrolled. Additionally, there were 14 672 special classes for mentally retarded children and 1142 special classes for speech-disordered children.

Starting in 1980, the JSCAP has engaged in activities to obtain official recognition of child psychiatry as a clinical departments, and themes regarding education in child psychiatry and child psychiatric medicine have been discussed at congresses and other such opportunities. The 12th Congress of the IACAPAP held in Kyoto in 1990 had a great impact in many respects, and there has been a rapid rise in interest regarding child psychiatry, which we take to be the greatest reward for having held the Kyoto Congress despite the many difficulties involved. Upheld by the success of that Congress, we were able to realize one of our hopes: the establishment of a system of designation and accreditation of child psychiatrists by the Japanese Society of Child and Adolescent Psychiatry.

Issues Regarding Training and Education

We have recently conducted a questionnaire survey of all medical schools and departments in Japan on postgraduate training in child psychiatry [3, 4]. The results show that many schools have a curriculum that includes 2 years of junior residency followed by 3 years of senior residency after graduation. Ninety percent of the schools believe it necessary to provide basic education in child and adolescent psychiatry within the framework of training for general psychiatry at some point within the 5 years, but only 60% of medical schools actually incorporate such a program.

We then conducted a survey on specialized training in child and adolescent psychiatry. Seventy-six percent of the schools believed that this education is necessary, but 19% believed it to be highly difficult at this time. Sixty-six percent noted that such specialized training should be carried out in each medical school, whereas 19% thought it was sufficient if such training were made available in one of three or four schools; 7% believed it should be delegated to specialized institutions outside medical schools. The duration thought suitable for such training was 1 year by 37%, 2 years by 29%, 3 years by 15%, and 4 years (or longer) by 11%. Nineteen percent of the schools had curricula for specialized training in child and adolescent psychiatry, and 48% did not. Reasons for not having such specialized curricula included lack of advisory staff, lack of specialized clinics or hospitalization facilities, lack of cases, lack of an adequate number of residents interested in specializing in this field, lack of sufficient financial backing by the university hospital, and uncertainty with regard to the future of child psychiatrists.

Taking such findings into consideration, I have tried to analyze why the number of institutions and specialists in child and adolescent psychiatry and the affiliated disciplines are not increasing in Japan as they should be [5-7].

1. The medical insurance system in Japan is such that just renumeration cannot be gained from the practice of child psychiatry, which has not been given official recognition as a clinical department. This lack of financial backing gives rise to continuous financial struggles.

2. With child and adolescent psychiatry not being taught as an independent subject in the university medical schools, training of specialists is insufficient. Hence cooperation with other clinical institutions in this area is difficult to establish, creating a vicious circle.

3. There are few positions available at the various medical institutions in Japan in which specialization in child psychiatry can be put to use.

4. A flaw in the training system of our schools of medicine is that positions as instructors or staff for training are not officially recognized.

5. There is a shortage of paramedical staff with clinical training, making it difficult to establish clinical teams. At present, there are no systems for training clinical psychologists, speech therapists, or psychiatric social workers, nor is there any system for their formal accreditation. Furthermore, there are no integrated systems for training specialized teachers to undertake special education, and it is not an exaggeration to say that the education of children with special needs is presently being upheld solely by the efforts of the individuals directly involved [8-11].

6. A shortage of nurses has become an important issue in Japan, and there is absolutely no system for training nurses specifically for child and adolescent psychiatry.

Such are the difficulties facing us, but the 12th Congress of the IACAPAP held in Kyoto in 1990 has given great momentum to our movement, and the importance and validity of child and adolescent psychiatry has come to be widely recognized by society. We are determined to continue our efforts at various levels for the establishment of child and adolescent psychiatry as an independent subject in medical schools and to gain official recognition as an independent clinical department.

References

1. Yamazaki K, Inomata J, Makita K, Mackenzie JA (1992) Japanese culture and neurotic manifestation in childhood and adolescence. In: Chiland C, Young JG (eds) New approaches to mental health from birth to adolescence. Yale University Press, New Haven, pp 384-391
2. Yamazaki K, Inomata J, Mackenzie JA (1987) Self-expression, interpersonal relations, and juvenile delinquency in Japan. In: Super CM (ed) The role of culture in developmental disorders. Academic, New York, pp 179-204

3. Hayashi M, Yamazaki K, Makita K (1985) Graduate and postgraduate education in child and adolescent psychiatry in Japan. Jpn J Child Adolesc Psychiatry 26:122–128
4. Makita K (1980) Graduate education in child psychiatry. Jpn J Child Adolesc Psychiatry 21:79–94
5. Honjyo S, Wakabayashi S, Sugiyama T, Otaka K (1985) Child and adolescent psychiatric education in Nagoya University. Jpn J Child Adolesc Psychiatry 26:128–135
6. Minagawa K (1985) Postgraduate education in child and adolescent psychiatry. Jpn J Child Adolesc Psychiatry 26:144–147
7. Shimizu M (1985) Graduate and postgraduate education in adolescent psychiatry. Jpn J Child Adolesc Psychiatry 26:139–141
8. Kado S (1985) Graduate education in child and adolescent psychiatry under liaison with pediatrics. Jpn J Child Adolesc Psychiatry 26:141–144
9. Murase K (1985) Graduate and postgraduate education of the clinical psychologist. Jpn J Child Adolesc Psychiatry 26:135–137
10. Ooi M (1985) Graduate education in child and adolescent psychiatry in the School of Education. Jpn J Child Adolesc Psychiatry 26:137–139
11. Takagi S (1980) Advice to specialists of child psychiatry and their co-workers. Jpn J Child Adolesc Psychiatry 21:95–103
12. Miyake K, and Yamazaki K (1995) Self-conscious emotions, child rearing, and child psychopathology in Japanese culture. In: Fischer K, Tangley J (eds) Self-conscious emotions: The psychology of shame, guilt, embarrassment, and pride. Guildford, New York, pp 488–504

Keyword Index

Author Index